Also by Win Tadd and by the same publisher

Ethics and Nursing Practice: A Case Study Approach (R. Chadwick and W. Tadd)

Ethical Issues in Nursing and Midwifery Practice: Perspectives from Europe (W. Tadd (edited))

Ethics in Nursing Education, Research and Management: Perspectives from Europe (W. Tadd (edited))

Ethical and Professional Issues in Nursing
Perspectives from Europe

Edited by

Win Tadd

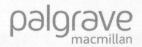

palgrave
macmillan

First published 2004 by
PALGRAVE MACMILLAN
Houndmills, Basingstoke, Hampshire RG21 6XS and
175 Fifth Avenue, New York, N.Y. 10010
Companies and representatives throughout the world

PALGRAVE MACMILLAN is the global academic imprint of the Palgrave
Macmillan division of St. Martin's Press, LLC and of Palgrave Macmillan Ltd.
Macmillan® is a registered trademark in the United States, United Kingdom
and other countries. Palgrave is a registered trademark in the European
Union and other countries.

ISBN 0–333–74993–6 paperback

This book is printed on paper suitable for recycling and
made from fully managed and sustained forest sources.

A catalogue record for this book is available from the British Library.

10   9   8   7   6   5   4   3   2   1
13   12   11   10   09   08   07   06   05   04

Printed in China

*Dedicated to the memory of my parents
Tom and Nancy Leonard – I owe them so much.*

Contents

Acknowledgements

I would like to express my deepest gratitude to all those who have helped me to complete this project. First I would like to thank the many nurses and health professionals whom it has been my privilege to know and work with in both the UK and Europe. I have learned so much through their willingness to share their thoughts and experiences – thank you.

I would also like to thank the contributors whose diligence and punctuality made my work as editor so much easier.

I also owe a debt of gratitude to the staff of Palgrave Macmillan, especially Jon Reed and Magenta Lampson, for their endless patience and constructive criticism.

Finally I would like to thank my husband, Vic, and my children, Rebecca and Andrew, for their love and support.

List of Table and Figures

About the Contributors

Peter Allmark is a lecturer in nursing at the University of Sheffield. He is a graduate in philosophy and completed his RGN at Oxford School of Nursing in 1986. He gained an MA in health care ethics at the University of Leeds in 1993 and recently completed his PhD at the same institution. His thesis is entitled 'An Aristotelian Approach to Informed Consent'. He was involved in a three-year multi-centre project, Euricon, funded by the European Commission, which examined informed consent and neonatal research. His nursing background is in general nursing, especially coronary care. He is married to Jacqui and has a son, Tom.

Marianne Arndt was until recently a lecturer in the Department of Nursing and Midwifery, Stirling University and Humboldt University, Berlin. She has published widely in nursing and nursing ethics and her research interests include ethics, gender studies and ethics education. She was a founder member of the International Centre for Nursing Ethics. With colleagues from Finland, Spain, Greece, Germany and the UK she has taken part in EU-funded collaborative research investigating issues of consent, privacy and autonomy in nursing interventions. Professor Arndt is now a candidate nun at the Kloster St Marien zu Helfta in Eisleben, Germany.

Andrew Edgar studied sociology and philosophy at Lancaster University and the University of Sussex. Since 1990 he has taught philosophy at the University of Wales, Cardiff. He became a member of Cardiff's Centre for Applied Ethics in 1990, and its director in 1993. Dr Edgar has published in a range of collections and journals, including *Bioethics* and the *Journal of Philosophy and Medicine*. He has participated in a number of European Commission funded projects on the allocation of health care resources, virtue ethics and chronic illness and dignity and older Europeans. He is co-author of *The Ethical QALY* (1998).

Georges Evers worked at the Centre for Health Services and Nursing Research, School of Medicine Catholic University in Leuven, Belgium.

He was also active in clinical nursing practice as a clinical nurse specialist in the multidisciplinary pain clinic of the University Hospital, Leuven. He also held a chair in clinical nursing research at the University of Witten Herdecke in Germany.

Georges Evers was born in the Netherlands, where he studied classics at Nijmegen University. He studied nursing in Nijmegen and earned his master's and PhD at Maastricht University Netherlands. He was Assistant Professor at the University of Maastricht for many years and worked for the Dutch National Council for Public Health as Chair of the Commission of Health Professions and as Chair of the Scientific Nursing Council of the Dutch Institution for Quality Assurance in Health Care. He moved to Belgium in 1990 and was active in Germany from 1997. Since 1999 he was involved in the European Network of Doctoral Education and in 2000 was made a Fellow of the European Academy of Nursing Science.

It is a great sadness that Georges died in June 2003. He will be missed greatly by nursing colleagues across Europe and the loss of his contribution to the profession will be felt for many years.

Maria Gasull is a registered nurse and midwife. She is Senior Lecturer at the Escola Universitaria de Infermeria Sant Pau, Universitat Autònoma de Barcelona in Spain and is an expert in bioethics (postgraduate course). Before entering nurse education she worked as a clinical midwife for ten years. She is a member of the Hospital Ethics Committee and member of the Advisory Comission of Bioethics for The Autonomous Catalonian Goverment. She is a member of the Editorial Board of the journal *Nursing Ethics*. Maria was the Spanish partner of a Biomed project, 'Patients' autonomy and privacy in nursing interventions', funded by the European Commission and coordinated by Helena Leino-Kilpi, University of Turku, Finland.

Søren Holm holds a medical degree, a degree in philosophy and religious studies, a PhD and a higher Danish medical doctorate (Dr. Med. Sci.), all from the University of Copenhagen as well as a master's degree in health care ethics from the University of Manchester. He has been teaching quantitative and qualitative research methodology and philosophy of science for many years, and has extensive experience of using qualitative research methodologies in health care settings. He has written papers on the philosophy of science of qualitative research, on continental philosophy as a resource for medical philosophy, and on health care ethics.

Dr Holm is currently Reader in Bioethics at the Institute of Medicine, Law and Bioethics of the University of Manchester and Professor at the Centre for Medical Ethics, University of Oslo. Every Tuesday he works in the ovarian cancer clinic in the Department of Medical Oncology at Christie Hospital, Manchester, where he is an honorary registrar.

Tom Keighley qualified in general, psychiatric and community nursing, and practised and taught in all three disciplines. In 1982, he joined the Royal College of Nursing as an adviser and became involved in national policy formulation. Between 1986 and 1993 he served on management boards at district and regional level. In 1993 he founded the Institute of Nursing at the University of Leeds and from 1996 to 2001 worked as Director of International Development in the School of Healthcare Studies. From 1989 to 2000 Tom served as the UK representative of the Practising Profession of Nursing on the Advisory Committee for the Training of Nurses in Brussels and continues to advise the UK government departments and the EU Commission on related issues. Since 1996 he has been editor of the journal *Nursing Management*. Also since 1996 he has served as a trustee on the board of St Gemma's Hospice. In 2001 Tom started offering freelance consultancy services to a range of health care, university and church/faith related organizations on a local, regional, national and international basis.

Reg Pyne has been a registered nurse since 1955. He had experience as a nurse in clinical and managerial posts before joining the staff of the former General Nursing Council for England and Wales and, from the date of its establishment, the United Kingdom Central Council for Nursing, Midwifery and Health Visiting. He was awarded a council of Europe Medical Fellowship in 1978/79, which was used to study the regulation of the nursing professions in European countries. His particular interests are the standards and ethics of professional practice legislation and effective professional regulation. He has written and spoken extensively on these subjects.

Reg's spare time is filled by activities in his local community, where he is Chairman of East Hertfordshire Community Health Council and the Secretary of the Amnesty International Group.

P. Anne Scott is Professor and Head of Nursing, Dublin City University. Her research interests include philosophy and ethics in health care and nursing practice, with special focus on autonomy, empowerment and virtue ethics; clinical judgement and decision-making; and the influence of humanities in health care practice. She is a member of the Editorial Boards of the *Journal of Nursing Philosophy* and the *Journal of Medical Humanities*. She has published widely in the areas of nursing ethics, philosophy and nursing practice.

Win Tadd is Senior Research Fellow in the Department of Geriatric Medicine, University of Wales College of Medicine. In 1989 she was made an International Fellow of the Hastings Center, New York, where she undertook research into nursing ethics, and in 1997 she was awarded a Fellowship by the UKCC to explore the use of the Code of Professional Conduct by UK nurses. She has published widely in the areas of health care and nursing ethics and her research interests include: ethical aspects of ageing and care of older people; quality of care; quality of life; professional ethics and research ethics. She is coordinator of an EU-funded project exploring dignity and older Europeans, co-coordinator of a second EU study exploring the information needs of older disabled people and a partner in a third European study exploring ethical codes in nursing.

1

Challenges and Issues in Nursing

Win Tadd

Introduction

This is the third volume in a series of three, exploring ethics and nursing from the perspective of the wider Europe. Volume 1 discussed the ethical aspects of nursing, with different client groups bringing to those discussions perspectives from various European countries. Volume 2 focused exclusively on the ethical aspects of nursing education, research and management, again bringing perspectives from a range of European countries. This volume will explore a number of issues that are of importance to the nursing profession in Europe.

When speaking of Europe, many people automatically think of the European Union, which has 15 member states and is preparing for the accession of another 13 eastern and southern European countries over the coming months. Europe's borders, however, extend far beyond those of the European Union. Europe includes over 50 countries, many languages, diverse cultures and values, together with more than 800 million people. It is not surprising, therefore, that in anticipation of changing geographical, political and social borders, the topic of globalization is one that attracts growing attention.

Globalization

Although there is much debate as to whether increasing globalization is a good or bad thing, it is undoubtedly a feature of twenty-first-century living, where time and distance no longer represent overwhelming obstacles. The world is a smaller place and we can no longer ignore what is happening in the lives of our global neighbours, be they in a near country or a far-flung continent. Their lives affect ours as people, goods, money, services, not to mention values, ideas and lifestyles move from one country to another, and few if any areas of our lives are immune to the effects of globalization.

Proponents of globalization suggest that it brings economic, social, political and health benefits, while antagonists argue that it increases exclusion and inequality, but what exactly do we mean by globalization?

Scholte (2000) argues that there are five common usages of the term. The first is 'internationalization' and refers to the cross-border activities and interdependence of countries. These increased transactions augment the effect that events and circumstances in one state have on others. Second, globalization is referred to as liberalization, as state-imposed restrictions on movement are either removed or reduced, resulting in what is often referred to as a borderless world economy. A third sense of globalization concerns universalization, where not only goods and services are available worldwide, but so too are ideas and experiences. Globalization is also connected with modernization, in particular changes which reflect western ideologies, and result in the spread of structures such as capitalism and industrialism to other cultures. Often the old and dominant values of these cultures and countries are destroyed or greatly modified in the process. Finally, Scholte claims that globalization can be described as deterritorialization or a transformation of geography. Although people generally differ in the emphasis they place on each of these aspects of globalization, she argues that it is this last aspect that is really new because, in so many areas of our lives, the world or global space is seen as a single entity and this reduces the importance of distance or national borders. These areas include, for example, finance, where billions of euros can be moved instantaneously from one country to another; communication, where via the Internet one can communicate cheaply and instantaneously with people halfway across the world; climate change brought about by the activities of some inhabitants of planet earth, which affects the whole world; and the movement of some 400 million people per year across national boundaries and vast distances, which can result in the spread of diseases from one continent to another within short periods of time. What impact, then, does globalization have on health care generally and nursing in particular?

Globalization, health care and nursing

The challenges to health care imposed by globalization are complex and cannot be fully addressed within the confines of this chapter, but citing some of these will demonstrate the complexity of the issues to be dealt with. In developing countries, infections and malnutrition, largely due to poverty, lead to most infant and maternal ill-health and mortality, and yet a relatively small contribution by the western world could virtually eliminate this.

Emerging epidemics, such as AIDS/HIV, will result in more than 20 million people being infected in the early part of the twenty-first century. In addition, by 2005, almost half of all AIDS cases may be caused by viruses resistant to treatment. The re-emergence of other epidemics such as malaria and drug-resistant TB will also challenge health systems across the world.

Environmental threats such as ozone depletion (mainly through the actions and lifestyles of people in developed countries) will result in increased health risks from skin cancers in other countries. Consumption of illegal drugs has increased ten-fold in the past 20 years, while tobacco use is rising, especially in the developing world, as US trade policy has resulted in governments relaxing restrictions on the trading of tobacco companies.

The increased movement of people will contribute to the international spread of infections and diseases. Although advancing technology will improve early detection, diagnosis and management of disease for many of the world's populations through the advent of telemedicine, for example, such technology is beyond the means and scope of many of the world's populations.

A report by the World Health Organization's Commission on Macroeconomics and Health (2001) estimated that 8 million lives per year could be saved in low-income countries by 2010 by increased investment and straightforward interventions. The interest of today's world leaders in health is being fuelled by a recognition that global health and security are 'inextricably intertwined' (Smith, 2002, p. 54) and investment in health is a vehicle for development. Their tardiness in this recognition is startling, bearing in mind that this was acknowledged in the nineteenth century: 'The health of the people is really the foundation upon which all their happiness and all their powers as a state depend' (Benjamin Disraeli, 1804–1881). Be that as it may, however, the claim is that saving lives and reducing ill-health will increase economic productivity, and few dispute that investment in health is essential for economic growth which would benefit both rich and poor countries alike.

As well as threats or risks to health raised by globalization, there are other dangers: poverty, inequality and increasing exclusion, to name a few. For example, world trade rules force small maize farmers in Mexico to compete with large-scale farmers in the US who benefit from large government subsidies, British consumers spend some £23 billion on clothes per year, (about Euros 650 per person) and yet workers producing the cotton or denim are probably paid less than Euro 1 per day. Indeed, 1.3 billion people survive on little over Euro 1 per day (Frenk and Gomez-Dantes, 2002).

A further threat of increasing globalization is the insensitivity to local cultures and the threat to cultural diversity, leading to at best intolerance and at worst conflict, xenophobia and ethnic cleansing (Frenk and Gomez-Dantes, 2002). This also provides the breeding ground for terrorism. Globalization therefore impacts on health and wellbeing generally and also on those who provide care, such as nurses.

Globalization and nursing

Nurses represent the escalating participation of women in skilled migration, and the situation in nursing is such that this topic was both the focus of debate at the International Council of Nurses Congress in Copenhagen in 2001 and the subject of a large international nursing conference in Atlanta in October 2001. The conference, 'Global Nursing Partnerships: Strategies for a Sustainable Nursing Workforce', involved representatives from governments and nursing associations, including government chief nursing officers, national and international nursing association leaders, and human resource directors/health planners from more than 60 countries (see http://www.nursing.emory.edu/LCCIN/EmoryHSNews.htm, 2001). Many countries, such as the UK, the Netherlands and Ireland, as well as those further afield such as Australia and America, have a shrinking nursing workforce as many nurses approach retirement themselves, which when coupled with the increased demands of ageing popula-tions, fewer recruits to the profession as a result of wage-based discrimination and high wastage rates (Hawthorn, 2001), has resulted in countries with severe nursing shortages increasingly relying upon international recruitment. For example, whereas Ireland was once a key exporter of nurses, it is now a significant importer and has a national strategy to deal with the acute shortages. Unemployed nurses from European countries such as Spain, Finland and Germany are targeted, as well as those from developing countries who can ill afford the leakage, such as the Philippines and South Africa.

Authough many countries have adopted policies to address the issues raised by severe nursing shortages, Buchan (2002) argues that any approach that focuses on the problem solely as a nursing problem is doomed to fail until chronic nursing shortages are addressed 'as a symptom of wider health system or societal ailments'. These 'ailments' include the undervaluing of nurses and nursing work, the restricted access to resources that nurses have, thereby reducing their effectiveness, a reluctance to address issues of health system and workforce planning, and restrictive professional role boundaries. One of the most deplorable aspects in relation to international recruitment, apart from robbing some developing countries of their much-needed nursing resources, is that many qualified nurses are faced with appalling periods in limbo before their qualifications are recognized and, when they are, their conditions of service often fall below those of 'home-grown' nurses.

While migration and international recruitment in nursing emerge as key issues in the globalization debate, they are not the only ones. Global acceptance of economically based imperatives of rationalization has resulted in convergence of education and health policies, and this has led to a growing number of international alliances in nurse education.

With increasing globalization, advances in communication and technology have meant that people from all corners of the world can be treated not only in their own community but also remotely through tele-medicine, and nursing has to be prepared for such technological advances.

Nurses, therefore, need to be culturally sensitive in their work and aware of the cultural and legal liabilities of working across national borders and in new settings. The Internet is probably the most evident example of globalization's impact on nursing practice as information, products and services reach people quickly and patients are frequently better informed, although misinformation is also a problem.

In addition, worldwide advertising campaigns and availability of information mean that people also tend to self-medicate more, especially with 'complementary' products that are less rigorously regulated.

Thus globalization is bringing improvements and dilemmas, and if nurses are to take full advantage, they need to be knowledgeable. Nursing research, for example, must address today's health care issues, such as the emerging and re-emerging infections mentioned above. Despite the increasing number of European and indeed internationally based educational programmes at both the under- and postgraduate level, nurse education must become more globally focused to ensure that nurses are better prepared to work with people from widely different cultures as well as in different locations. Although increasingly nurses are competing successfully for European and international research funds, for example Leino-Kilpi recently coordinated a study into autonomy in nursing practice in three countries, van der Arend is currently coordinating a study into codes of nursing ethics in seven countries[1], and Tadd is coordinating a multiprofessional project across eight centres into dignity and older Europeans (see www.cordis.lu for further information), more needs to be done to ensure widespread dissemination of both information and findings to enable other nurses to benefit from such multicultural experience and research.

As emphasized in both previous books in this series, the aim of the series is to stimulate and encourage dialogue and debate among European nurses so that we can collaborate and learn from each other in ways that will benefit not only nurses, but also patients, clients and the population as a whole. Never has the need for this been greater than now.

The rest of this book

This aim of this book is to consider some of the key professional issues facing European nurses. It begins in Chapters 2, 3, 4 and 5 by exploring those issues that face the nursing professions across Europe. Chapters 6, 7 and 8 focus more intently on issues affecting individual practice, such as interprofessional collaboration, professional autonomy and the nurse's role as patient advocate. In Chapter 9 the gap between the more general professional issues and those affecting the individual is bridged by an exploration of nurses' ethical codes and finally, in Chapter 10, the issues involved in nurse regulation are addressed.

In Chapter 2 Evers explores the diversity that exists in European nursing. In doing so he address differences in statutory regulation, nursing education and in the division of labour in the nursing workforce. Evers also comments on the similarities and trends in nursing roles across Europe. In particular he examines the benefits and drawbacks posed by increased nurse specialization and the advent of the nurse practitioner role, before considering some key challenges that nurses in Europe will need to face in coming years. Not least of these is the lack of power that nurses generally experience. However, escalating health costs, an ageing population, technological advancement and widespread cultural changes will also challenge Europe's nursing profession. To meet these challenges, Evers argues for the need for evidence-based nursing practice and a well-educated workforce led by competent, skilled clinical leaders to ensure provision of effective and efficient patient care.

Søren Holm, in Chapter 3, addresses one of the key issues for nursing raised by evidence-based practice. This is the apparent demand for 'hard' quantitative data on which to base care decisions. This he states is an issue for nursing because major parts of nursing research in non-quantitative and certain nursing theories appear to be antithetical to evidence-based practice. He begins by exploring the motivation and justification for evidence-based practice. Following this, Holm explores the differences between research that is relevant to evidence-based practice and that which is not. However, he is careful to emphasize that simply because a study is irrelevant to the evidence-based practice agenda, this is not to say that it is not important research.

Holm goes on to examine the contributions that qualitative studies can make to the progress of evidence-based practice. Two examples appear of particular importance here. The first is where the outcomes of a specific intervention best suit an investigation using qualitative methods, for example when trying to gauge complex effects such as changes in quality of life, or when an outcome may be quantifiable but its intensity can only be determined by qualitative methods, for instance, the impact of organizational change or education.

An important thread which Holm addresses at length is the seeming obsession that some qualitative researchers have with positivist approaches to research, and he argues that over-concentration on the differences hides the fundamental similarity in inferential procedures of both approaches. He also criticizes the apparent obsession with the claim by some proponents of the qualitative paradigm that it is essential to master the philosophical underpinnings of their various research methodologies, arguing that for the most part, this is virtually impossible for those not trained in philosophical methods. Also he emphasizes that most people rely on secondary sources rather than original texts in their attempt to achieve this aim. To highlight the dangers of this practice, Holm uses the example of Heidegger's work. A good qualitative study, claims Holm, will not be judged by its philosophical underpinnings, but by the rigour with which it is performed.

Chapter 4 explores the role of nurses in European health policy development. Tom Keighley begins by emphasizing that Europe is in a constant state of flux and that determining any profession's role is necessarily difficult because of national variations in the professional structures, education and preparation for leadership. He begins his analysis with a brief historical account to show the fluctuating nature of Europe's internal boundaries and how some influential nursing groups came into being. Keighley goes on to examine the development of the European directives on general nursing and the mutual recognition of nursing qualifications before describing the work of the WHO Europe and its attempts to ensure that nurses are educated to meet the health demands of the twenty-first century. Like Evers, Keighley considers the impact of specialist nurse education in Europe and the drive to ensure that nursing adopts a strong research base. Like Evers, Keighley recognizes that the greying of the European population means that the demand for nursing services will grow, and because of improved access to information the population will be better informed than ever before of health care options. The changes, he argues, increase the need for a highly educated nursing workforce.

In terms of nursing practice impacting on policy development, Keighley explores the work of a number of European nursing networks such as the European Oncology Nursing Society, but he warns that the rise of such specialist groups may fragment the National Nursing Associations and thereby reduce their effectiveness on the European front. Enlargement of the Union and organizational changes in the EU itself also present significant challenges for Europe's nurses. Finally Keighley emphasizes the importance of lobbying to influence the European health agenda in Europe, encouraging nurses to use the resources of their national organizations to ensure their impact is felt.

Marianne Arndt continues with the political threads discussed in Keighley's chapter by addressing whether political activity is a professional duty of nurses. She begins by examining the relationship between politics and ethics, arguing that nursing ethics needs to be viewed from three different perspectives, the political or macro perspective, the institutional perspective and finally the personal. Arndt argues that although the hallmark of excellent nursing practice is at the point of direct care, the 'not-free-to-be-moral' debate must be taken into account. The issues about personal and professional autonomy and accountability raised by this debate are further examined by Scott in Chapter 7. Arndt goes on to examine the role of various nursing organizations, statutory and professional, in the UK, Germany, Austria and Switzerland. The role of these organizations is explored in relation to their political activity and involvement, and then from the perspective of educational advancement in nursing. This chapter throws light on how difficult some of the calls for improved education made in Chapters 2 and 4 are in practice.

Multidisciplinary teamworking is a feature of health care in many European countries. In Chapter 6, Maria Gasull explores what is involved in effective teamwork, beginning with the characteristics of a profession, before considering the much-cited doctor–nurse game first coined by Stein. She explores research studies on doctor–nurse relationships before identifying the prerequisites of successful interprofessional working. This she argues ultimately depends on the moral attitudes of team members, particularly those of respect, trust and responsibility.

In Chapter 7 Anne P. Scott addresses the question which Gasull takes for granted, namely whether nurses are autonomous professionals or subservient workers. She begins by giving a detailed account of autonomy, exploring its relationship to freedom, accountability and responsibility. After considering whether full autonomy is a possibility for anyone, Scott explores autonomy in the context of today's nurses, distinguishing between moral and professional autonomy and highlighting the effect that systems can have on one's experience of it. She argues that to be autonomous professionals nurses must acquire professional maturity and be willing to accept professional responsibility, particularly for exercising moral autonomy in the course of their work.

A common expectation of the nursing role in many European countries is that nurses will act as the patient's advocate and plead their cause when necessary. Peter Allmark addresses some of the issues surrounding this role and asks whether nurses in fact have any special claim to fulfil it. He explores the emergence and development of the advocacy movement before suggesting that one major source of confusion is the nature of the cause that the nurse is meant to plead. A second source of confusion is the particular type of advocacy that is expected. The inherent confusions which arise from the various causes and types of advocacy mean that nurses can sometimes find themselves having to plead opposing causes. The major problem that results is one due to proponents and opponents of the role talking at cross-purposes. Allmark suggests three possible resolutions to these issues before proposing that the term be dropped from the nursing vocabulary and a different model of ethical conduct adopted.

The issue of ethical conduct in nursing is explored further by Andrew Edgar in Chapter 9 on codes of nursing ethics. He provides and examines examples from a number of nursing codes. According to Edgar the majority of these codes frequently fail to achieve their intended outcomes because they fail to satisfy certain conditions of readability. Problems of interpretation and ambiguity further hamper the effectiveness of many codes, as they fail to provide nurses with a framework to reflect upon and make sense of their moral conduct. Edgar shows the characteristics of effective codes and argues strongly that codes which set out to provide a set of practice guidelines fail because they do not bridge the gap between general principle and the particular situation faced by practitioners. For codes to be useful moral documents they must challenge nurses to reflect upon what it means to be a professional nurse in the unique situation in which they find themselves.

The final chapter by Reg Pyne explores the topic of professional regulation in Europe, focusing on the challenges increasingly mounted in relation to professional regulation. He then examinies five key principles which need to underpin any system of professional regulation. He closes by challenging all nurses to consider whether their regulatory system is sufficiently robust to ensure that the public interest is safeguarded.

It is hoped that the contributions in these pages will not only stimulate nurses to think about some of the key issues in their professional lives, but also encourage them to debate the issues with colleagues and fellow professionals across Europe. Only through such dialogue can the problems and challenges facing nursing and nurses be addressed in ways that will enhance their practice and ensure their patients receive the high-quality care they deserve.

Note

1. Helena Leino-Kilpi (Finland), together with nursing colleagues in Spain, Greece, Germany and UK coordinated a Biomed 2 project 'Patient's *autonomy* and *privacy* in nursing interventions' funded by the European Commission. Arie van der Arend is coordinator of a European project 'Ethical Codes in Nursing'. For further information see {HYPERLINK 'http://www.zw.unimaas.nl/ecn/'}

References

Buchan, J. (2002) 'Global nursing shortages', *BMJ*, 324: 751–752.
EMORY Health Sciences News (15 November 2001) Robert W. Woodruff Health Sciences Center Emory University http://www.nursing.emory.edu/LCCIN/EmoryHSNews.htm
Frenk, J. and Gomez-Dantes, O. (2002) 'Globalisation and the challenges to health systems', *BMJ*, **325**: 95–97.
Hawthorn, L. (2001) 'The globalisation of the nursing workforce: barriers confronting overseas qualified nurses', *Australia Nursing Inquiry*, **8**: 213–229.
Scholte, J.A. (2000) 'Globalisation, governance and corporate citizenship', Third Annual Warwick Corporate Citizenship Unit Conference, Scarman House, University of Warwick 10 July.
Smith, R. (2002) 'A time for global health', *BMJ*, **325**: 54–55.
WHO (2001) *Macroeconomics and Health: investing in health for economic development*, Report of the Commission on Macroeconomics and Health, Geneva: WHO.

2

The Nurse's Role – Present and Future

Georges Evers

Introduction

All European health care systems face fundamental changes and, as a consequence, the role of nurses is being challenged in all European countries. This challenge includes increasing both the effectiveness and efficiency of nursing care while preserving its compassionate and human character.

Summary

This chapter will explore the diversity in European nursing in terms of legal regulation, educational programmes, distribution of nurses and the division of labour. The chapter will also explore common characteristics of the nursing role within European health care systems. The merits and disadvantages of increasing nurse specialization and nurse practitioner roles will also be considered. At the end of the chapter possible future developments will be discussed.

Diversity in European nursing

Legal regulations

The picture of nursing in Europe is rather diverse and complex. First, the 'picture' depends on what is meant by Europe. If one takes the perspective of the World Health Organization, the landscape stretches from the shores of the Atlantic Ocean in the west to the Ural Mountains in the east and from the North Pole to the Sahara Desert in the south. If one takes the borderlines of the Council of Europe, we speak about nursing in 40 different countries in the north, west, east and south of Europe. If the borders of the European Union are used, then European nursing differs between Austria, Belgium, Denmark, Finland, France, Germany, Greece, Ireland, Italy, Luxembourg, the Netherlands, Portugal, Spain, Sweden and the United Kingdom. For the purposes of this chapter, Europe will be defined in this way.

The picture of nursing in Europe is diverse because Acts governing nursing practice differ in the various countries of the European Union (Versieck *et al.*, 1995). In Germany and the Netherlands the practice of nursing is not legally protected, but use of the title 'nurse' is protected by law. In Germany this means that nursing tasks can be performed by anybody, not only by 'nurses'. On the other hand, not everybody is allowed to use the title 'nurse' (Krankenschwester/-pfleger), 'paediatric nurse' (Kinderkrankenschwester/-pfleger) or 'second-level nurse' (Krankenpflegehelfer/-in). To use these titles, a person has to apply for clearance, which can only be obtained under the following conditions:

- if the person has followed an educational programme and passed the final state examination;
- if the person can demonstrate that he/she has no physical or psychological frailty, addiction and has not shown any behaviour that would make it impossible to enter the nursing profession.

Nurses are not obliged to register in Germany when they want to practise. A similar system of title protection is regulated by law in the Netherlands, while the practice of only a limited number of medically prescribed nursing activities, considered to be dangerous for the patient, is protected by law.

In other EU countries the practice of nursing is legally protected (Versieck *et al.*, 1995). In Belgium, regulations of nursing practice are established by the federal government and only persons holding certain titles are legally allowed to practise. To be able to practise within the profession, individuals must apply for written authorization (right to practise) to the Provincial Medical Commission, which is a division of the Ministry of Public Health and Environment. After verifying qualifications the Medical Commission issues the authorization and registers the nurse.

In Denmark those wishing to nurse must have a general diploma in nursing and apply for registration with the National Board of Health, which is related to the Ministry of Health. In France nurses are obliged to register their qualifications at the Provincial Health Service in one of the 21 regions in which they work, and they should register anew when they go to work in another region. In Greece there is a law regulating licensure through which both the nursing title and practice are protected. The licence is issued by the 'prefect' or state official of the area in which the nurse wants to work. In Ireland every student who completes the recognized nurse education programme must register with An Bord Altranais so that their name can be placed on the active register maintained by this body. The functions of An Bord Altranais include the registration of the nurses, the regulation of their education as well as professional conduct and fitness to practise.

In Italy only persons who are in possession of the state diploma of 'Infermiere Professionale' are legally allowed to practise nursing. Nurses who want to practise must register. The registration is run by the Federatione Nazionale dei Collegi IPASVI on a provincial basis. This national federation is also responsible for the protection of the nursing profession and for disciplinary actions when the code of conduct is contravened. In Luxembourg registration as a professional, the practice of nursing and re-registration are regulated by legislation introduced in 1992. In Portugal nursing diplomas must be registered before entry into the profession. Registration is supervised by the Ministry of Health and takes place in the Regional Health Administrations. Nursing diplomas obtained outside Portugal must be registered in the Department of Human Resources of the Ministry of Health. A licence document (Carteira Profissional) given by the Ministry of Employment and Social Security, which includes the professional title of nurse (Enfermeiro), is needed to work in public and private institutions and also to work on a self-employed basis.

In order to practise nursing in Spain it is necessary to have obtained the Diplomado en Enfermeria and to register with the professional organization of Colleges of Nurses in the province where one wants to practise. All provincial Colleges of Nurses are grouped in the General Council of Nursing Colleges. In the United Kingdom all nurses, midwives and health visitors are required to have effective registration with the Nursing and Midwifery Council (NMC). The Council determines the entry requirements and the kind, standards and content of training and education programmes needed for admission to the register. The Council also evaluates applications from persons qualified abroad who seek registration. Further, it provides advice on professional conduct, determines whether practitioners should be removed from the register and prosecutes those who falsely represent themselves to be qualified or registered.

Educational programmes

Nursing within the EU also differs in respect of entry requirements concerning minimum age, such as 16 to 18 years, and levels of secondary education vary for the different types of nursing programmes. Basic educational programmes can differ in level and length, for example, the Belgian A1 professional and A2 vocational/technical programme, or the Dutch nursing and caring educational programmes, which are on five qualification levels. Formal second-level nurse education programmes exist in Germany, Greece, Italy, Luxembourg, the Netherlands and Spain. Educational programmes for other caring personnel exist in Belgium, Denmark, Germany, Greece, Italy, Luxembourg, the Netherlands and Portugal.

Basic educational programmes can also differ in their focus, such as preparation for general nursing only, as in Denmark, France, Greece, the Netherlands, Portugal and Spain. They may also prepare specialized nurses, such as those working in paediatrics, gerontology or psychiatry/mental health, in addition to general nurses, as in Germany, Italy, Ireland, Luxembourg and the United Kingdom.

Midwifery is considered to be a specialization within nursing, as basic nursing education is required, in Ireland, Luxembourg, Portugal and Spain, while in Belgium there is one year of common education. In Denmark, France, Germany, Greece, Italy, the Netherlands and the United Kingdom midwives are educated in separate educational programmes. In most countries nurses are granted some reduction in the length of the midwifery programme. Operating theatre and radiological nursing are considered as specialist areas in some countries, such as Belgium, while separate educational programmes are organized in other countries, such as the Netherlands, for operating theatre or radiology technicians.

Basic nursing education can be totally included in the university system, as in Finland, Portugal, Spain and the United Kingdom, partly included, as in Greece or Italy, or be in the non-university sector, as in Belgium, Denmark, Greece and the Netherlands. In some countries, such as Austria, Germany and France, nurse education is in the secondary technical or vocational education sector. Basic nursing education can be regulated by hospitals, as in Germany, be under the jurisdiction of the Ministry of Health, as in France, or under the jurisdiction of the Ministry of Education, as in Belgium.

Since 1977 minimum standards for the education of professional nurses have been developed and implemented in the European Economic Community (EEC), the European Community (EC) and later the European Union (EU). These standards concern 'nurses responsible for general care' having completed a basic general training of at least three years. This has made freedom of movement possible for general nurses in the 15 member states of the EU. Directives 77/452/ EEC, 77/453/EEC, 77/454/EEC, 77/455/EEC, 89/595/EEC spell out the following minimum standards:

- a general school education of ten-years' duration attested by a diploma, certificate or other formal qualification;
- full-time training, of a specifically vocational nature, which must cover the subjects of the programme set out in the annex of the directive;
- programmes must constitute a three-year course or 4,600 hours of theoretical and practical instruction;
- the length of the theoretical instruction shall amount to no less than one-third and that of clinical instruction to no less than one-half of the minimum length of training;
- theoretical instruction is provided by teachers of nursing and other authorized persons and is delivered in nursing schools and other places chosen by the schools in which education is provided;
- clinical instruction is provided in hospitals, other health care institutions and in the community under guidance of nurse teachers and in collaboration with and with the assistance of other qualified nursing personnel.

In a similar way the following midwifery directives have been developed and implemented: 80/154/EEC, 80/155/EEC, 80/156/EEC and 80/157/EEC (Quinn, 1982; Verieck *et al.*, 1995).

In conclusion, nurses with the following categories of educational programmes may practise within the EU (Versieck *et al.*, 1995): general nurses with a diploma in accordance with EU nursing directives; nurses with a basic specialist education; nurses other than general nurses, who have received basic education in a specialty and are equipped to work only in this specialty; and second-level nurses (that is, nurses with a basic general education shorter than three years). In addition, categories of caring personnel who do not qualify as nurses may practise within the scope of nursing. The scope of practice of caring personnel can overlap with nurses' tasks, as seen for instance in care of older people. The scope of certain paramedic technicians in some EU member states may also overlap with nurses' tasks in other states.

Distribution of nurses

The total number of active registered general nurses with a diploma in accordance with EU directives within the European Union can be estimated at about 2.4 million for 373.9 million inhabitants (see Figures 2.1 and 2.2). This estimation has been calculated on available

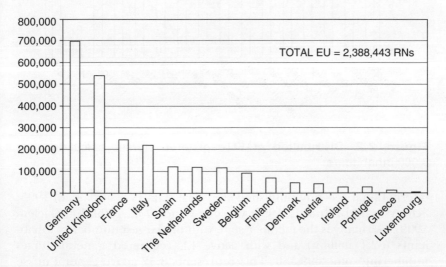

Figure 2.1   Distribution of EU-registered nurses in absolute numbers

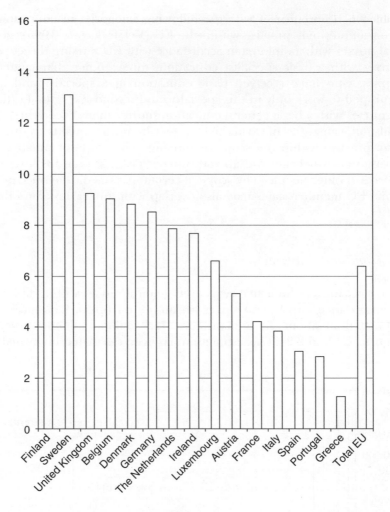

Figure 2.2 Distribution of EU-registered nurses calculated per 1,000 inhabitants

international recently published statistical data (Versieck *et al.*, 1995; Schutyser and Edwards, 1999; van der Windt *et al.*, 1999; Van Tielen, 1999). Germany is the member state with the largest number of inhabitants (82.1 million) and with active EU-registered general nurses numbering some 699,580. This represents 8.52 active general nurse per 1,000 inhabitants. Luxembourg is the member state with the smallest

Table 2.1   Distribution of EU-registered nurses among EU member states

EU member states	Inhabitants (millions)	Active registered nurses	EU-registered nurses (per 1,000 inhabitants)
Austria	8.1	42,930	5.3
Belgium	10.2	91,965	9.02
Denmark	5.3	46,791	8.83
Finland	5.1	69,870	13.7
France	58.5	246,071	4.21
Germany	82.1	699,580	8.52
Greece	10.6	13,407	1.26
Ireland	3.7	28,406	7.68
Italy	57.4	220,702	3.84
Luxembourg	0.4	2,642	6.6
The Netherlands	15.4	120,000	7.86
Portugal	10.0	28,380	2.84
Spain	39.7	120,251	3.03
Sweden	8.8	115,280	13.1
United Kingdom	58.6	541,168	9.23
Total EU	373.9	2,388,443	6.39

Sources: Versieck *et al.* (1995); Schutyser and Edwards (1999); van der Windt *et al.* (1999); Van Tielen (1999).

number of both inhabitants and active EU-registered nurses (2,642), representing 6.6 active general nurses per 1,000 inhabitants. For the EU as a whole this figure is 6.39 active general nurses per 1,000 inhabitants. Table 2.1 shows a considerable variation between member states in the proportion of active EU-registered general nurses per 1,000 inhabitants. The figure is lowest for Greece (1.26) and Portugal (2.84) and highest for Finland (13.7) and Sweden (13.1).

When these figures are compared with the percentage of gross domestic product (GDP) in euros (€) spent on health care per capita in the different member states, no relationship can be detected. Germany (10.4 per cent) and France (9.4 per cent) spend most, while Denmark (5.5 per cent), the United Kingdom (5.7 per cent) and Ireland (5.8 per cent) spend the least. The member states with the lowest numbers of registered nurses per 1,000 inhabitants, Greece (1.26) and Portugal (2.84), together with those with the highest numbers, Finland (13.7) and Sweden (13.1), spend comparable percentages of their GDP on health care: 8.0, 8.2, 7.6 and 7.6 per cent respectively.

When the figures are compared with the distribution of medical doctors per 1,000 inhabitants, again no clear relationship can be detected. Spain (4.2) and Germany (3.4) have the highest number of medical doctors per 1,000 inhabitants, while Ireland (0.8), Denmark (0.89) and Italy (0.9) have the lowest numbers (Schutyser and Edwards, 1999). The respective distribution of active EU general nurses in these member states is 3.03, 8.52, 7.68, 8.83 and 3.84 per 1,000 inhabitants. Portugal and Sweden have an identical (3.2) proportion of medical doctors per 1,000 inhabitants, but they score at the extremes in the distribution of active EU general nurses with 2.84 and 13.1 per 1,000 inhabitants respectively. Germany (3.4) has by far the most general medical practitioners per 1,000 inhabitants and Greece (0.1), the United Kingdom (0.6) and Sweden (0.6) the least. The distribution of active EU general nurses for these member states is 8.52, 1.26, 9.23 and 13.1 per 1,000 inhabitants.

Division of labour

In all European Union member states most nurses are employed in health care institutions. But the percentage of registered general nurses in relation to the total number of hospital employees in full-time equivalents differs greatly. This figure is 17 per cent in Portugal while it is about 45 per cent in Ireland, Belgium and the United Kingdom. In France the proportion of nursing costs in relation to the total hospital budget is lowest at 19 per cent, whereas in the United Kingdom and Luxembourg it is highest, accounting for some 45 per cent (McKenzie, 1991; Evers, 1992, 1993, 1997). The number of active second-level nurses varies also. Germany (122,500), Spain (91,568), France (61,000), the Netherlands (56,000), Italy (53,356) and Denmark (48,000) employ the most. The United Kingdom employs by far the most registered nurses with specialist basic education (227,160) (Versieck *et al.*, 1995). The proportion of nurses employed in health care institutions as opposed to self-employed, or employed in community or home care also differs across European Union member states.

Interpretation of all the above figures should be undertaken with caution. National statistics are obviously not equally reliable and comparable, but the overall conclusion is clear. These figures indicate diversity in the division of labour, in delineation of responsibilities and tasks of EU general nurses both within health care institutions and between these institutions and the community. They indicate diversity in delineation of responsibilities and tasks compared to medical doctors, paramedical technicians, second-level nurses and other caring personnel (both qualified and volunteers) and family members of patients. They also indicate diversity in nurses' contributions to health promotion, disease prevention, recovery, rehabilitation, and palliative and terminal care.

Diversity in division of labour implies different combinations of nursing and other tasks and different role sets. Nursing tasks can be divided into the following categories: preventive, educative, caring, supportive, diagnostic, therapeutic, coordinating, reporting, administrative and housekeeping tasks (Bakker and le Grand van den Bogaard, 1992; Bouten *et al.*, 1995). Preventive tasks include the following:

- surveillance and detection of patients or groups of patients at risk from preventable disabilities, handicaps, impairments, complications and diseases;
- early detection of signs and symptoms;
- patient reactions to disease, handicap or treatment.

Educative tasks include the following:

- providing information, advice and instruction to patients or patient groups about nursing care techniques and procedures;
- providing health education to patients or groups of patients;
- providing information and instruction to patients and patient groups in diagnostic and treatment procedures;
- providing information about institutional procedures;
- providing information about patients' rights and obligations within health care institutions (Evers, 1999).

Caring tasks include providing assistance with activities of daily living: bathing, dressing, eating, drinking, elimination, mobility and transfer. Supporting tasks include the following:

- listening and approaching patients with respect, understanding, empathy and personal involvement;
- providing emotional support; stimulating patients to find their own solutions;
- providing comfort measures and reducing discomfort;
- providing a safe, clean and 'therapeutic' environment.

Diagnostic and therapeutic tasks include the following:

- performance of routine diagnostic and treatment procedures;
- collection of diagnostic samples;
- first aid;
- administration of oxygen, parenteral fluids medication;
- insertion and removal of naso-gastric and bladder catheters;
- application of warmth and cold; wound care (Evers, 1999).

Coordinating tasks include:

- designing and implementing individual nursing care plans;
- patient allocation or task allocation;
- delegation and supervision of nursing activities;
- consultation or referral to colleagues and other health professionals.

Reporting and administrative tasks include the following:

- participation in nursing and multidisciplinary team discussions about patients;
- reporting and documenting facts, observations and impressions about patients and their nursing and medical treatment plan.

Housekeeping tasks include:

- distributing meals;
- making beds;
- cleaning and maintenance of medical and nursing appliances and apparatus;
- keeping the living environment of patients clean (Evers, 1999).

Diversity in division of labour also implies differences in role sets of nurses (Evers, 1992, 1993). The following roles have been identified:

- nature's helper in restoring the body to health;
- a mother substitute/the professional mother;
- the physician's assistant in caring for the ill and preventing disease;
- the physician's complement – the physician concentrating on cure, the nurse on care;
- a substitute for the physician;

- a coordinator of the services of all health workers;
- a manipulator of the environment;
- a trainer and director of personnel with less preparation;
- a health educator;
- someone who, through the nursing process, enables the client or patient to make the best use of health resources;
- someone who applies 'nursing science' for the betterment of mankind;
- someone who intervenes on the client's or patient's behalf in a crisis or time of need;
- the patient's and family's helper in meeting their health needs (Henderson and Nite, 1978).

These roles are not mutually exclusive and are usually combined into various role sets.

Common characteristics of the nursing role

Despite this diversity in legal regulations, educational programmes, distribution of nurses and division of labour, some important common role characteristics can be identified. In all European Union health care systems nursing plays a pivotal role. Nursing's main function in all these health care systems is to guarantee organizational permanency in meeting the basic human needs of the patients (Evers, 1997). Therefore, nursing's role is pivotal for the smooth running of health care systems. This function was and still is rooted in basic moral and social values of the common European cultural heritage that stem from the unique combination of the Judaeo-Christian and the Graeco-Roman traditions.

In the Judaeo-Christian tradition of 'caritas', feeding the hungry, sheltering the homeless, nursing the sick and injured and comforting the hopeless were highly valued. In the Graeco-Roman tradition of 'humanitas', respect for the individual person, human dignity and the right to be free, even of discomfort and disease, were highly valued. Nursing in Europe was born in the Judaeo-Christian tradition of 'caritas'. Compassion, respect and solidarity with the weak and persons in need were and still are the central values of our profession. These values are also the backbone of any health care system in the European Union. And they have shaped nursing's unique function in European society (Evers, 1997).

This societal function of nursing has been accurately and clearly defined by Virginia Henderson. She identified this function as being:

> To help people, sick or well, in the performance of those activities contributing to health or its recovery (or to a peaceful death) that they would perform unaided if they had the necessary strength, will or knowledge. It is likewise the function of nursing to help people gain independence as rapidly as possible. (Henderson, 1966, p. 4)

In addition or as part of this defined function, if it is broadly interpreted, nursing's aim is to help patients carry out therapeutic plans as initiated by physicians (Harmer and Henderson, 1955; Henderson and Nite, 1978). This societal function of providing a substitute for what patients lack to make them independent within the health care system has been further explicated by Dorothea Orem (1959, 1980, 1995) as compensation for inabilities in self-care or care for dependants and as education in and support of self-care or dependent care. This compensation, education and support is described as the planned and coordinated use of helping methods such as doing things for, or collaborating with patients and their families, providing information, advice or training and providing material, emotional or environmental support.

Inabilities in self-care or problems with self-care ('self-care deficit') can be described as assessment, decision or performance problems. These problems may have to do with supply of basic personal needs, 'universal self-care requisites'; with intelligent participation in medical diagnosis and treatment, 'health deviation self-care requisites'; or promotion of personal development and wellbeing, 'developmental self-care requisites'. Supply of basic personal needs includes: sufficient intake of air, water and food; body hygiene and elimination of excrements; a balance between activity and rest and between solitude and social contacts; prevention of falls, trauma, infection, intoxication, suffocation, colds and burns; and support from a social network (Evers, 1994, 1998).

Intelligent participation in medical diagnosis and treatment includes detection of symptoms such as fever, persistent coughing, irregular pulse, blood in the urine, white stool, green phlegm or irregular nodes in the breast and such-like; seeking and securing appropriate medical assistance from a physician, nurse, dietitian, physical therapist, social worker, for example; and to carry out medical prescriptions effectively. These might involve muscle exercises, blood glucose monitoring, wound care, intermittent bladder catheterization, colostomy care, or peritoneal dialysis; to monitor treatment effects such as weight loss, polyuria, hypoglycaemia, bleeding, pressure sores and the like; to control symptoms such as pain, vomiting, dyspnoea, itching and dry mouth; to make necessary changes in self-image with amputation, stoma, alopecia, organ transplantation, device implantation, prosthesis, or wheelchair dependence; and to make necessary changes in lifestyle such as diet change, smoking reduction, changes in leisure pursuits, or increasing social relations and so on (Evers, 1998).

Promotion of personal development and wellbeing includes mitigation of damage caused by loss of body parts or body functions such as paralysis of extremities, loss of the partner, parents, children, beloved personal belongings or a 'home'. This also includes mitigation of damage due to neglect such as emotional neglect of children, material neglect of parents, permanent contempt, physical abuse or rape. Promotion of personal development implies undisturbed transition to a next life episode or stage such as teenager, parent, retired or aged person, despite disease or treatment (Evers, 1994, 1998, 1999). The function of nursing in society is to compensate, educate or support when assessment, decision or performance problems occur in the above-mentioned domains of self-care or care for dependent persons.

A second and important common characteristic of the role of nursing is that it is largely performed by females. Nursing is a predominantly female profession in all European Union member states, although there is some variation in the female domination. In Greece the percentage of male general nurses is the lowest, at 2 per cent. Greece is followed by Denmark with 3.3 per cent, Italy with 5 per cent, Ireland with 6.5 per cent and France with 7 per cent. The United Kingdom and Germany follow with 12 per cent and 12.8 per cent respectively. Spain, Luxembourg and Belgium have 14 per cent, 14.3 per cent and 14.6 per cent male nurses in the general sector. The Netherlands (15.3 per cent) and Portugal (16 per cent) have the largest proportion of male general nurses (Schutyser and Edwards, 1999).

As a predominantly female profession nursing plays a pivotal role, but one that is not in the spotlight. The role is usually played without being noticed, without acknowledgement. Women are cordial, nice and warm. Of course they are also intelligent, but, strictly speaking, not intelligent enough for really important decisions. This gender issue in the stratification of medical and nursing roles in the health care systems has been described as the 'doctor–nurse game'. One of the best descriptions of this game was that of Stein (1967) (see Chapter 6 by Maria Gasull this volume). He was fascinated by the strange way in which nurses made recommendations to physicians, observing that they pretended they had not done so. Physicians, in turn, pretended that nurses never made recommendations. Yet Stein noted that the more highly regarded physicians were careful to follow nurses' recommendations. He called the pattern a transactional neurosis. It seems to be an exaggerated version of the traditional male–female game in which relatively powerless females gain power over males by manipulation. It is supported by reciprocal systems of reward and punishment, as well as by tradition. Most nurses are apparently unconscious of the game, yet they play it well and have been conditioned to do so throughout their professional lives. Unfortunately for patients, however, the communication pattern of the game is not efficient. Crucial information is lost or its transmission slowed so that patient care suffers and the dignity of both the nurse and physician roles is reduced (Bullough, 1978).

The really important decisions in health care are medical and economic ones. Nursing, patients and society as a whole are caught in these stereotypes and public debate and political decision-making about nursing are conditioned. Yet the reality of everyday practice is different from the stereotypes. On a daily basis nurses make many decisions that are crucial for the recovery and maintenance of functional abilities, for safety, comfort and tolerance of both patients and their families. But these decisions are insufficiently defined, recognized or rewarded. In everyday practice, nursing is usually responsible for the way medical and economic decisions are implemented in patient care. Very often the patient, together with the nurse, is the first to experience the practical consequences of these decisions. Yet the way in which most public debates about health care reforms take place is based primarily on stereotypes about nursing and not on the reality of everyday practice. Nursing's voice is hardly heard, let alone reflected in the media, and it is missing at many levels of strategic decision-making. When it is heard it invariably lacks sufficient power and impact (Evers, 1997).

The challenge

Nursing is the largest professional group within all the health care systems in the European Union. The common backbone of all these

European health care systems is solidarity with the weak and those in need. Health care systems in Europe can be classified as based on either the social health insurance model, the so-called Bismarck system, or the National Health Service model (Ham, 1997; Lenaghan, 1997). In 1883 Bismarck initiated a statutory health insurance system 'Gesetzliche Krankenversicherung' in Germany. Initially it included only blue-collar workers, which resulted in 10 per cent of the population being eligible for health care coverage. Over the last hundred years, more and more sections of the population were included in the health insurance. In parallel, the benefit package became gradually more comprehensive (Busse *et al.*, 1997). The other EU member states with social health insurance are Austria, Belgium, France, Luxembourg and the Netherlands. The social insurance model covers 90 per cent of the population in Germany, 60 per cent in the Netherlands and *de facto* the whole population in Austria, Belgium, France and Luxembourg. The six countries use different terms to define the group of insured persons. Austria, France and Luxembourg have universal coverage for their social health insurance system, Belgium also has universal coverage but applies a two-tier system, one for the employed with a large benefit package and one for the self-employed covering only major risks. In Germany a large proportion of the population has mandatory insurance, with a small portion legally excluded. This leaves a third group of mainly employed people with incomes above a certain limit having a choice between statutory and private health insurance. The Netherlands has a system with universal coverage, first compartment (Exceptional Medical Expenses Act), and a second compartment with a strict separation between statutory and private health insurance along an income line. That is, there is no choice between the two systems, while a third compartment follows the rules of a market model.

In all six countries providers are a mix of public, not-for-profit and private status, but all are separated from the payers. In all countries except Germany the sickness funds are supplemented by a national umbrella organization, which is responsible for collecting and allocating contributions (Belgium, Luxembourg and the Netherlands) and/or paying hospitals (Austria and Luxembourg). Thus funds are the collectors of contributions in Austria, France and Germany and the actual payers in all countries except for hospital care in Austria and Luxembourg. Generally financing in all these countries relies mainly on income-related contributions. But there are important differences.

There is an upper limit on contributions in Austria, Germany, Luxembourg and the Netherlands, while there is no such limit in Belgium and France. The contribution rate is uniform in Belgium, France, Luxembourg and the Netherlands, while rates differ between funds in Austria and Germany. In Belgium, France and Luxembourg sickness funds receive quite substantial additional income through general taxation, and in Austria hospital care is mainly financed through taxation. Traditionally, physicians' services in all Bismarckian countries are paid on a 'fee-for-service' basis with the Dutch general practitioners receiving capitation payments as the exception.

Due to the ever-present payer–provider split, contracts have a long tradition in all Bismarckian systems. The scope of the contracts varies, however. In Belgium, France and Luxembourg, the specific benefits are defined by the various governments, leaving only service numbers and prices to the contract partners. In Germany the detailed benefits package, the level of reimbursement and the size of total reimbursement are negotiated. In the Netherlands selective contracting has been encouraged since 1992.

The other EU member states follow the National Health Service model. The distinctive features of its 'classical' form are:

- financing mainly by taxes;
- classical state administration;
- hierarchical allocation of resources;
- very often a separation between health care financing and provision;
- mostly no explicit benefit categories and no explicit rights for patients who are denied services;
- limited choices for the patient in selecting a provider.

Two subgroups of EU member states can be identified within this model: the so-called Beveridge group consisting of the British Isles and the Nordic countries, and the southern European countries consisting of Portugal, Spain, Italy and Greece, which changed from social health insurance systems to tax-based systems around 1980. In the first group changes were introduced during the 1980s and 1990s to make the system more efficient, competitive and responsive to consumers. The typical modification caused by the reforms in the 1990s in the Beveridge group and later in the southern European group is a separation between financing and provision. The best-known example is the so-called purchaser–provider split introduced into the United

Kingdom National Health Service by different forms of contracting with hospitals and other providers, although changing government policy has recently reduced this separation.

During the last two decades the moral and social value of solidarity has come under greater pressure in both models of health care systems of the EU member states. Since the beginning of the so-called crisis of health expenditure in the 1970s, cost-containment operations have been launched (Mossialos and LeGrand, 1999). In both models health care budgets were used as an attempt to control costs, and in the 1990s competition and market principles were introduced in various degrees in both models. Elements of the market model can be found in almost every European country. Its principles are most explicit in the private health insurance arrangements that cover more than a third of the Dutch and almost 10 per cent of the German population. Visible signs of convergence of the market model with the social insurance model are mandatory insurance, risk-independent premiums and collective negotiated contracts. The purchaser–provider split and the growing importance of health care entitlements are visible signs of convergence of the National Health Service model with the social health insurance model. Both systems face similar conflicts between solidarity and competition.

Both systems also face a financial crisis. The higher the number of unemployed and retired people, the narrower the financial basis of the system because of lower insurance contributions or tax revenues. Second, labour is responsible for an ever-decreasing share of the national income, while the share of capital is increasing. These factors result in a relative reduction of the financial flow to the insurance system since contributions are based only on labour. In addition, the so-called Maastricht norm, introduced to converge the different economies of EU member states to a monetary union resulting in the euro (€), put serious pressure on public spending in the 1990s. As far as nursing is concerned there is a third 'pressure' factor in relation to coverage of the benefit package.

Demographic (ageing of the population), technological (new treatment options) and cultural (reduced social support, social isolation, increased consumerism and patient rights) changes have led and will continue to lead to an increasing demand for nursing care. At the same time, health services are confronted by limited resources and budgetary restrictions. Both patients and nurses experience pressures of increased demand and intensity of need. This pressure is expressed as scarcity and the issue of distributing scarce time, attention and competence: 'Sorry, but we don't have time.' The pressure is also related to the issue of costs and reimbursement: 'Sorry, but we don't have money for that.' The pressure is also related to more fundamental shifts in the European cultural heritage from the Judaeo-Christian pillar of solidarity and altruism to the Graeco-Roman pillar. This is expressed in growing hedonism, individualism and group egotism: 'Sorry, but we don't have time and money for you.'

In times of fundamental revision of basic values and structures it is of utmost importance to be aware of the central values of the health care system and nursing's pivotal role in it. Health care without compassion and solidarity, without respect and attention for the physical, psychosocial and spiritual needs of patients and clients is not a quality health care in Europe. Quality health care in Europe cannot exist without quality nursing care. Nursing and society as a whole in Europe are confronted with a great challenge, which is to increase both the effectiveness and efficiency of nursing while maintaining a humane, caring service. Nursing's pivotal role should be improved and better explicated by the development of evidence-based nursing care. To put this simply, we must ask the following questions:

- Do we accurately identify persons who need and can benefit from nursing care?
- Do we concentrate our efforts on these persons in order to avoid both over-consumption and under-utilization of nursing care?

Too much or wrongly delivered nursing care will result in unnecessary dependence and handicap for the patients, unnecessary care burdens for the family and unnecessary costs for society. Too little or incompetent nursing care will result in unnecessary discomfort and suffering, unsafe conditions and unnecessary complications, morbidity and mortality for the patient, unnecessary care burdens for the family and unnecessary costs for society (Evers, 1997).

Evidence-based nursing and clinical leadership roles

This challenge is much more complicated than simply increasing the size of the nursing army. Society needs evidence-based nursing care. Reliable and valid data are needed about what we actually do in nursing to serve the needs of our patients. This scientific knowledge base can be generated by research on the incidence and prevalence of nursing problems/diagnoses and nursing-specific outcomes, and by research on frequency, effectiveness and costs of nursing interventions (Evers, 1997). Nursing problems/diagnoses can be classified as self-care problems or problems of health care delivery to dependent persons, that is, inabilities in self-care or inabilities in dependent care assessment, decisions or performance in the domain of supply of basic personal needs, intelligent participation in medical diagnosis and treatment or personal development and wellbeing. This classification fits with the disabilities section of the International Classification of Impairments, Disabilities and Handicaps (ICIDH). The primary responsibility and focus of the medical role and function in society is reflected in the International Classification of Diseases (ICD), the classification of Mental Disorders (DSM) and the impairments section of the ICIDH. Nursing interventions can be classified as total or partial compensation for inabilities in self-care/dependent care; teaching and counselling about self-care/dependent care; providing material and emotional support for self-care/dependent care; and providing a safe and stimulating environment for self care/dependent care. Nursing-specific outcomes can be classified as survival indicators, functional health state indicators, wellbeing, comfort, discomfort/distress reduction indicators, growth and development indicators. Scientific nursing knowledge refers to all possible relations between problems, interventions and outcomes and the relations with relevant variables in the environment. Scientific knowledge encompasses factual knowledge gained by research and clinical practice and understanding by speculative theories (Evers, 1997).

In order to meet the challenge of evidence-based nursing care, this knowledge base must also be applied in clinical practice. A number of barriers can be identified in relation to the profession of nursing, the practice of which historically had religious origins. Our culture is rather conservative, ritualistic and conformist. Nursing's structure is of a traditional and bureaucratic nature, often resulting in the ineffective use of nursing competence. Nursing leaders rarely remain in clinical practice and usually have no hard statistical data with which to negotiate and influence public debate and political decision-making. Nursing in practice is predominantly based on tradition and rituals and insufficiently based on scientific evidence. This is not to say that nursing should be purely scientifically based. Nursing was, is and always will be an art, like medicine. But this art deserves a better base than unchallenged rituals and tradition (Evers, 1997).

In order to develop this professional evidence-based nursing role, the education of 'officers' for the nursing army is critical for all European Union member states. In the present 'crisis' our efforts need to be concentrated on recruitment, selection and education of an elite group of talented youngsters for clinical leadership roles in nursing. The aim is to prepare students for clinical and managerial nursing leadership roles in health care systems which focus on decentralization and forms of managed care, case management and clinical pathways. Also, students need to be prepared for research-based practice in health care systems that focus on quality services, that is, on effective and efficient patient care.

Apart from increased effectiveness through evidence-based nursing, clinical leadership roles must also contribute to the efficiency of health care systems. Efficiency is the production of a given effect with the least cost or the greatest result within a specific amount of resources. A functional division of labour is crucial to goal achievement within any health care system, and in an effort to deal with the problem of escalating labour costs a differentiation of the nursing role has occurred. Within health care institutions much of the work of the nurse has been delegated to less expensive workers. The role has been fragmented into at least three levels: nursing aides, second-level nurses/practical nurses/caring professionals, as well as registered nurses. The quick fix of replacing registered nurses with less qualified health care providers has fragmented patient care and frustrated registered nurses, who in turn tend to leave the hospital service. Thus, to a large extent, nurses are aware of the negative consequences of role differentiation for patient care. The role of the registered nurse has changed from that of direct patient care provider to one of coordinator, administrator or technician. As a consequence nurses are being urged to 'come back to the bedside', to improve patient care and to expand the nursing role (Bullough, 1978). To operationalize this suggestion, the extended role of clinical nurse specialist has been developed. Clinical nurse specialists are nurses who have undergone advanced educational preparation, often at university level; they give expert care to seriously ill patients, act as role models, disseminate the scientific knowledge base into nursing practice and spend time with patients and families who need additional emotional support (Hardy and Conway, 1978). The clinical nurse specialist role emerged in response to the recognized need to improve the quality of patient care and the clinical practice of nursing, primarily in the acute setting (Henrick and Appleyard, 1997). Expert clinical practice is the *sine qua non* of the clinical nurse expert. Practice, that is the actual ongoing experience with patients and families, provides the content and directs participation in various sub-roles such as clinical research, consultation, teaching and leadership (Hamrick and Spross, 1989). Clinical nurse specialists work primarily in institutional settings, typically in staff positions. Regardless of organizational placement, the clinical nurse specialist usually works from a 'home base' and is available for consultation from other units. An important characteristic is the emphasis on improvement of the nursing function. Clinical nurse specialists are 'nursing's precious resource' (Henrick and Appleyard, 1997).

Differentiation of the medical role has also resulted in the development of both the nurse practitioner and physician assistant roles. Again the basic driving force behind this differentiation is an economic one, so that nurse practitioners have solved the problem of shortage of people who can deliver safe, efficient primary care at a reasonable cost (Bullough, 1978). Nurse practitioners are educated to perform a broad spectrum of primary care interventions, including health assessment, risk appraisal, health education and counselling, diagnosis and management of acute minor illnesses and injuries, and management of chronic conditions. They tend to perform as generalists rather than as specialists in terms of clinical practice, and one major concern is whether nurse practitioners function as physician substitutes or as nurses (Henrick and Appleyard, 1997; Barton *et al.*, 1999). If they function merely as physician substitutes they are a valuable contribution to the efficient performance of the medical function in society. But caring and curing are not mutually exclusive concepts. Rather, they are part of a continuum, and both physicians and nurses undertake health care activities in these arenas. Both caring and curative activities are necessary in primary interventions and can be combined in the nurse practitioner role. As far as there is sufficient emphasis on, and professional autonomy for, the nursing function, this expanded role is a valuable contribution to the nursing function in society. Thus there are more similarities than differences between the roles of clinical nurse specialist and nurse practitioner, with both roles being referred to as advanced practitioners (Forbes *et al.*, 1990).

Potential future developments

In a time of rapid change it is almost impossible to predict the future. The only valid prediction that can be made with confidence is that change will take place in nursing's role within Europe. The following changes are taking place at the moment and will probably influence nursing in all member states of the European Union. Hospitals will be further downsized; ambulatory care and home care will be expanded; more registered nurses will be replaced by less qualified personnel; enrolment in nursing programmes will continue to decrease; computers will be used more extensively, with increasing recognition of the need for a standardized nursing language for documentation purposes; concern with costs and delivery of a quality product will continue; concern will grow with regard to the care of the older people and those with chronic illnesses; and more patients and consumer groups will be included in health care policy-making and health politics.

Conclusion

Despite the many changes, the dilemmas will remain much the same as in the past. These include solidarity or individualism/group egotism, quality versus cost, safety versus risk, collaboration versus competition, dependence versus independence, unity versus diversity and standards versus access (Comi-McClosky and Kennedy, 1997). As in the past, in this new century, nursing and society will need leaders with a clear vision who are armed with hard statistical data for public debate and political negotiation about nursing's pivotal role in the health care systems in Europe.

References

Bakker, J. and le Grand van den Bogaard, M. (1992) *Dutch Social Policy Statement on the Nursing Profession*, Zoetermeer: National Council for Public Health.

Barton, T., Thome, R. and Hoptroff, M. (1999) 'The nurse practitioner: redefining occupational boundaries', *International Journal of Nursing Studies*, **36**: 57–65.

Bouten, R., Versieck, K., Pacolet, J. and Hedebouw, G. (1995) *Manpower problems in the nursing/midwifery profession in the EC*, Volume 2, Leuven: Hoger Instituut voor de Arbeid.

Bullough, B. (1978) 'Stratification', in: Hardy, M. and Conway, M. *Role theory: perspectives for health professionals*, New York: Appleton-Century-Crofts, pp. 157–177.

Busse, R., Howorth, C. and Schwartz, F. (1997) 'The future development of the rights based approach to health care in Germany: more rights or fewer?', in Lenaghan, J. (ed.) *Hard choices in health care – rights and rationing in Europe*. London: BMJ Publishing Group, pp. 21–47.

Comi-McCloskey, J. and Kennedy, G.H. (1997) *Current issues in nursing*, 5th edition, St Louis: Mosby.

Evers, G. (1992) 'Anforderungen an die Lehrer qualification in den Pflegeberufen im Hinblick auf den europäischen Binnenmarkt nach 1992', *Deutsche Krankenpflege Zeitschrift*, (9): 14–17.

Evers, G. (1993) 'The European experience of cancer nursing: curriculum development and dissemination', *European Journal of Cancer Care*, **2**: 29–33.

Evers, G. (1994) 'Orem's self care concepts of nursing practice', in Mashaba, T. and Brink, H. *Nursing Education: an International Perspective*, Cape Town: Juta and Co.

Evers, G. (1997) 'The Future Role of Nursing and Nurses in the European Union', *European Nurse*, **2** (3): 171–181.

Evers, G. (1998) 'Die Selbstpflegdefizit-Theorie von Dorothea Orem', in Osterbrink, J. (Hrsg) *Erster internationalen Pflegetheorieen Kongres Nürnberg*, Bern: Hans Huber Verlag, pp. 104–133.

Evers, G. (1999) *Theorieën en Principes van Verpleegkunde*, 3rd edn, Leuven/Assen: Universitaire Pers Leuven/van Gorcum.

Forbes, K., Rafson, J., Spross, J. and Kozlowski, I. (1990) 'The clinical nurse specialist and nurse practitioner: core curriculum survey results', *Clinical nurse specialist*, **4**: 63–66.

Ham, C. (ed.) (1997) *Health care reform: learning from international experience*, Buckingham/Philadelphia: Open University Press.

Hamrick, A. and Spross, J. (1989) *The clinical nurse specialist in theory and practice*, 2nd edn, Philadelphia: Saunders.

Hardy, M. and Conway, M. (1978) *Role theory: perspectives for health professionals*, New York: Appleton-Century-Crofts.

Harmer, B. and Henderson, V. (1955) *Textbook of the principles and practice of nursing*, New York: Macmillan.

Henderson, V. (1966) *The Nature of Nursing: A definition and its implications for practice, research and education*, New York: Macmillan.

Henderson, V. and Nite, G. (1978) *Principles and Practice of Nursing*, New York: Macmillan.

Henrick, A. and Appleyard, J. (1997) 'Clinical nurse specialists and nurse practitioners: who are they, what do they do, and what challenges do they face?', in Comi-McCloskey, J. and Kennedy, Grace H. *Current issues in nursing*, 5th edn, St Louis: Mosby, pp. 18–25.

Hospital Committee of the European Community (1993) *Hospital Services in the E.C.*, Leuven: Ceuterick.

Lenaghan, J. (1997) *Hard choices in health care – rights and rationing in Europe*, London: BMJ Publishing Group.

McKenzie, D. (1991) 'A review of nursing manpower issues', *Acta Hospitalia*, (2): 51–55.

Mossialos, E. and LeGrand, J. (eds) (1999) *Health care and cost containment in the European Union*, Aldershot: Ashgate.

Orem, D. (1959) *Guide for developing curricula for the education of practical nurses*, Washington: US Government Printing Office.

Orem, D. (1980) *Nursing: Concepts of Practice*, New York: McGraw-Hill.

Orem, D. (1995) *Nursing: Concepts of Practice*, St Louis: Mosby.

Quinn, S. (1982) 'Nursing education in the countries of the European Communities', in Henderson, M. (ed.) *Nursing education*, Edinburgh: Churchill Livingstone.

Schutyser, K. and Edwards, B. (1999) *Hospital Health Care Europe 1999/ 2000. The official HOPE reference book*, London: Campden.

Seymour, J. (1990) 'European round up', *Nursing Times*, **86** (48): 38–41.

Stein, L. (1967) 'The doctor–nurse game', *Archives of General Psychiatry*, **16**: 699.

Van Tielen, R. (1999) *Compendium Gezondheidsstatistiek*, Brussels: BIGE.

Versieck, K., Bouten, R., Pacolet, J. and Hedebouw G. (1995) *Manpower problems in the nursing/midwifery profession in the EC*, Volume 1, Leuven: Hoger Instituut voor de Arbeid.

Windt, W. van der, Calsbeek, H. and Hingstman, L. (1999) *Verpleging en Verzorging in kaart gebracht*, Maarsen, Utrecht: Elsevier/De Tijdstroom.

3

Evidence-Based Practice – The Role of Nursing Research

Søren Holm

Introduction

In recent years we have seen an ever-increasing emphasis on evidence-based practice (EBP) in health care. It started with evidence-based medicine in 1992, but has since spread rapidly to all other professions and parts of the health care system (Evidence-based medicine working group, 1992). The central claim of the EBP revolution has been that no intervention in the health care system should be performed and/or paid for unless we have good evidence that it is:

1. effective, and
2. at least as effective as the available alternatives.[1]

The fact that we have always treated or cared for our patients in a certain way is not a good reason to continue to do so. This demand for evidence of effectiveness is often converted into demands for properly conducted research with hard quantitative endpoints and later systematic reviews of all the available studies.

Institutions like the Cochrane collaboration, which coordinates the production of systematic reviews, together with the National Institute for Clinical Excellence in the United Kingdom (UK), which guides the National Health Service regarding the introduction of new treatments and the phasing out of obsolete treatments, are part of the EBP movement (Burke, 1999).

Within nursing, EBP initially seems to raise some problems because (1) major parts of nursing research are not quantitative, and (2) some kinds of nursing theory seem to be antithetical to EBP. I will leave the last problem to the professional nursing theorists, to whom I will also leave the problem of whether there is a general theory–practice gap in nursing, whether this matters, and what effects EBP will have on it (Upton, 1999).

Summary

The purpose of the present chapter is therefore to look more closely at the role of non-quantitative research in generating evidence and/or knowledge for EBP. The chapter begins by outlining the rationale for the introduction of EBP. This has partly been due to the recognition that theoretically sound interventions do not always work in practice and that what in the past may have counted as 'evidence' may not only be unreliable, but also harmful. Other drivers of EBP include the need to control escalating health costs and the moral obligation of professionals to demonstrate the soundness of their knowledge claims.

The chapter goes on to clarify the distinction between research that is relevant to EBP and that which is not, arguing that both categories may be equally important, before exploring how qualitative studies can contribute to EBP. Following this, the apparent conflict with positivist research methods to which qualitative researchers frequently allude is considered and suggestions are made to reduce this divide. Using the example of phenomenology, it is then shown that the differences in epistemological and philosophical underpinnings do not necessarily invalidate the EBP movement, before highlighting the dangers of relying on secondary or tertiary philosophical literature to support various qualitative methodologies. Instead it is concluded that rigour and methodological soundness will determine the value of qualitative research and, provided these are met, qualitative studies have much to offer evidence-based practice.

What is the rationale for the 'evidence-based' revolution?

The idea that health care practice should be evidence based is obviously not new. From the first emergence of non-religious healing practices, practitioners have claimed to have a solid knowledge base for their various interventions. This has always been a combination of theories about the workings of the body and empirical observation of the effects of various interventions. The balance between the perceived importance of theory and observation has continually changed over time and each major paradigm shift in medicine has led to the emergence of both new theories and new observations.[2]

In the last century we have experienced a tremendous growth in our theoretical knowledge about the functions of the human body and mind as well as in our empirical knowledge about the effects of various influences on them. Through the last century, too, there has been a movement towards making increasingly stringent demands concerning the quality of the evidence for the effectiveness of various interventions, and EBP is just the latest incarnation of these demands (previously we have, for instance, had much the same in the form of 'clinical epidemiology' or 'rational medical decision-making').

Why has this happened? One reason is that experience has shown that many interventions with a good theoretical rationale do not work when they are implemented in practice and their effectiveness is assessed. Many interventions which theory predicts should work and which work in animal experiments do not work in clinical practice. Sometimes it is possible to find an explanation for this failure and sometimes it is not. This possible disjunction between theoretically predicted effectiveness and actual effectiveness means that it is very risky to implement interventions in clinical practice purely on the basis of theory. Some evidence that it actually works in the way intended is needed.

To say that we need more evidence than that provided by theoretical prediction, however, is still not to say very much. Evidence comes in many forms. If I say that I applied psychological technique P to further the grieving process of one of my patients, and that the patient then grieved appropriately, it is evidence that P works, but not very strong evidence. The movement we have seen through the last century has been from an acceptance of uncontrolled evidence ('I treated X patients and Y became better'), over a requirement for unsystematic controlled evidence, for example, historical evidence ('This year I treated X patients and Y became better; last year when I still used the old method, only Z became better'), to a requirement for well-controlled evidence, such as evidence from a randomized, double-blind, controlled trial.

This move towards greater and greater demands concerning the way evidence is generated has again been occasioned by the realization that some of the older ways of generating evidence are inherently unreliable and may lead us to believe that a certain intervention is effective in cases where it is actually harmful. The problem that EBP tries to solve, that is, the uncontrolled introduction of untested health care interventions and the persistence of old obsolete interventions, is one that all the health care professions have to take seriously.

If we look at the process in epistemological terms, we are, over the years, simply requiring better epistemic warrant for our knowledge claims about the usefulness of an intervention.[3] There are also external factors that have influenced the call for more and better evidence. One of these is the realization that rationing is inevitable in any health care system. It seems sensible first to try to rationalize the current system by removing interventions that do not work and in the future only to introduce interventions that do work. At the same time politicians want more control over spending on health care, together with more accountability from professionals, and the EBP movement promises to deliver on all these counts (O'Reilly, 1997).

A second external factor is the increasing focus on ethics in the health professions. People come to health care professionals for care, treatment and advice because they believe that health care professionals possess a certain kind of knowledge. This creates an ethical obligation on the professions to make sure that their knowledge claims are actually well founded. It is ethically problematic to intervene in people's lives unless we know that our interventions are likely to help them.

EBP and research practice

The rationale behind EBP points to certain kinds of research being relevant and other kinds of research being irrelevant, and for our purposes here, it is important to be clear about exactly where this dividing line is placed and what it actually means. The placing of the dividing line will be the topic for the next section, after we have considered the meaning of the divide. In both of these analyses it is, however, important to keep two things apart:

1. the requirements that follow from the underlying rationale of EBP; and
2. the claims and statements made by unreflective practitioners of EBP.

These are very different things. There is no doubt that many EBP practitioners put forward inflated claims about the importance of EBP, as well as not sufficiently thought through and rather bombastic methodological and practical advice. Much of this is, however, not derivable from the underlying rationale (Sackett *et al.*, 1996; Feinstein and Horwitz, 1997).

The major textbook on evidence-based medicine defined it in the following way:

> Evidence-based medicine (EBM) is the integration of best research evidence with clinical expertise and patient values.
>
> - By *best research evidence* we mean clinically relevant research, often from the basic sciences of medicine, but especially from patient-centered clinical research into the accuracy and precision of diagnostic tests (including the clinical examination), the power of prognostic markers, and the efficacy and safety of therapeutic, rehabilitative, and preventive regimens. . . .
> - By *clinical expertise* we mean the ability to use our clinical skills and past experience to rapidly identify each patient's unique health state and diagnosis, their individual risks and benefits of potential interventions, and their personal values and expectations.
> - By *patient values* we mean the unique preferences, concerns and expectations each patient brings to a clinical encounter and which must be integrated into clinical decisions if they are to serve the patient. (Sackett *et al.*, 2000, p. 1)

Within the EBP framework, research is relevant if it aims to add to the evidence base concerning the effectiveness of one or more health care interventions. Research is irrelevant if it has other aims, or if it is of such poor quality that it cannot add to the evidence base. Based on a pragmatic analysis of the costs and benefits of various kinds of research, it can further be seen that in choosing between different research designs one should choose the design that is most likely to provide an epistemically well-justified answer to the research question. In many cases this will be some version of controlled trial, but this is not always the case. For an intervention to be EBP-assessable it minimally needs to have one or more specified aims, and the achievement of these aims, must be capable of investigation by some kind of research methodology.

But what about research that is not EBP-relevant? Is it bad or unnecessary research? No, definitely not. The distinction between what is EBP-relevant and EBP-irrelevant is simply a distinction between research relevant in a specific context and research not relevant in that context. The rationale behind EBP does not entail that only EBP-relevant research is important. It is quite conceivable that some kinds of basic research that are not directly EBP-relevant may be extremely important because, for instance, they lead us to revise our theories or develop totally novel theories.

An uncontroversial way[4] to fit qualitative research into the EBP framework is thus to use it in the hypothesis-generating phase of research (in Popperian language in the 'Context of discovery' instead of in the 'Context of justification'), or as pilot studies prior to the deciding quantitative studies. This uncontroversial way of accommodating qualitative research is, however, also fairly uninteresting. In the next section we will try to explore whether a role can be found for qualitative research within the core EBP enterprise.

Evidence and qualitative research[5]

It is evident that the EBP movement primarily focuses on quantitative research, with hard outcomes as the 'best' type of evidence for the effectiveness of a given intervention, and this seems to leave qualitative research out in the cold as far as EBP is concerned. This situation is further complicated by the fact that some qualitative researchers claim to belong to a different research paradigm than the paradigm held by quantitative researchers. The paradigm problem will be discussed in the next section; here we will primarily consider whether there might not be room for qualitative research within the EBP framework after all.

As mentioned above, an intervention can be assessed within the EBP framework if it has one or more defined aims whose achievement can be assessed via some kind of research method, and further that the best available research method should be chosen. This excludes from the EBP framework those kinds of research where the main purpose is to understand why something happens, what motives the agents involved have and such-like. If the following definition of qualitative research in a standard textbook on nursing research were valid, it would exclude most if not all qualitative research from the EBP context:

> Qualitative analysis is concerned with describing the actions and inter-actions of research subjects in a certain context, and with interpreting the motivations and understandings that lie behind those actions. (Porter, 1996, p. 330)

But the definition is clearly too restrictive. If, for instance, I perform a qualitative study of the quality of life of persons with diabetes, the study falls outside Porter's definition if my main aim is to understand the psychological elements that together add up to 'quality of life'. This example also indicates a possible role for qualitative research within EBP. For certain health care interventions the desired aims are not direct changes in 'objective' health status but changes in quality of life, self-perceived health, social adjustment or one of many other similar outcomes.[6] There have been many attempts to measure outcomes like these quantitatively, but they are characterized by considerable controversy. If we, for instance, look at the quality-of-life literature it is immediately evident that there are large differences in the definitions of the central concept and, therefore, great differences in the various proposed measures (Griffin, 1986; Bowling, 1997). It may therefore be the case that an intervention primarily aimed at quality-of-life improvement could most appropriately be assessed using a qualitative methodology for the assessment of the outcome, that is, a change in quality of life. This could be done in a pre-/post-design, or as part of a randomized study. Similarly, an intervention aimed at changing the nurse–patient interaction in a specified way could conceivably best be assessed using qualitative analysis of participant observation data.

What these examples indicate is that qualitative research could more generally have a role within the EBP framework if it could be shown that there are certain kinds of relevant outcomes of health care interventions that are best assessed using qualitative methodologies. If that is the case, the rationale behind EBP would not only leave room for qualitative research; it would actually require it to be used in appropriate circumstances.

Can something more be said about what kind of outcomes we are talking about here? The desired outcomes of the interventions in the examples given above seem to be characterized by two common features:

1. they are not biological; and
2. they are multi-faceted and unlikely to be reducible to some enumerable set of measurable features.

It is important to note that it is not the case that the outcomes cannot be measured now, but may become measurable sometime in the future, but that we have good reasons to believe that no quantitative measuring device will ever be able to measure the outcome in a fully comprehensive, and thereby satisfactory, way.

A second core role for qualitative research within the EBP framework will be in those cases where the outcome is quantifiable, but where the actual 'intensity' of the intervention can only be appropriately gauged by qualitative methods. This will be the case for a number of interventions involving organizational change, education or training, or personal development.

Qualitative research and positivism bashing

A specific feature of the qualitative research methodology literature is that a significant proportion consists of writings on the basic philosophy (of science) of this kind of research. Methodology books often contain fairly lengthy chapters on this issue and there are many, many books and journal articles specifically concerned with it (see for instance Polkinghorne, 1983; Kvale, 1989; Morse, 1994). This is in sharp contrast to the quantitative methodology literature, where one seldom finds such chapters, and where discussion of the underlying philosophy (of science) is most often relegated to specialized philosophy journals. A recurrent motif in the qualitative literature is the ritual condemnation of positivism and all its evils and deeds. The Other (the medical researcher?) is a positivist but we (the enlightened?) have moved beyond this stage.[7]

This is often combined with a rejection of 'ontological realism' either for social reality or for reality *tout court*, and the adoption of some form of social constructivism (Guba and Lincoln, 1998). If social constructivism is accepted in its strongest form as the underlying philosophy for qualitative research in the health care field, it follows fairly straightforwardly that there is no place for qualitative research within the EBP framework. Basic terms within that framework like 'intervention', 'outcome' and 'effectiveness' would simply no longer have any determinate meaning, and the qualitative researcher would have excluded him or herself by rejecting the basic rationale for the whole EBP enterprise. This would, for instance, be the case if we accepted the view put forward by Gergen and Gergen in an (in)famous paper from 1991:

> The confirmations (or disconfirmations) of hypotheses through research findings are achieved through social consensus, not through observation of the 'facts'. The 'empirical test' is possible because the conventions of linguistic indexing are so fully shared ('so commonsensical') that they appear to 'reflect' reality. Thus, for example, we can treat the proposition 'John was in class this morning' as empirically verifiable because the meaning of the terms of the proposition are so broadly shared that they seem to be 'mirrors' of the world . . . Thus, whether or not John was *actually* in class depends on what one is willing to call 'John', 'class', 'in' and the like and not on what is given to observation. (Gergen and Gergen, 1991, p. 82, emphasis in original)

It is true in a very trivial sense that whether or not John was actually in class depends on the meanings of the words in the proposition, but from this trivial observation about propositions it does not follow that whether John was actually in class depends *only* on these linguistic features. Gergen and Gergen invalidly infer the false conclusion '*x* is *only* dependent on *y*' from the true premise '*x* is dependent on *y*'. Even a fully competent member of the English linguistic community could not tell us whether John was in class this morning without access to some observational data.

It can more generally be shown that social constructivism is a highly implausible and probably self-defeating position with regard to physical reality but a more plausible, although not philosophically compelling, position with regard to social reality (Collin, 1997). This leads to an important query with regard to qualitative research in the health care field. On what side of the physical reality versus social reality divide do our research projects fall? If our projects fall on one side of the divide and the projects that form the background of prominent qualitative research methodologists fall on the other side of the divide, we may be misled by their strong social constructivist leanings, which may not be applicable to our projects. To posit a simple physical–social reality dichotomy is a gross simplification since many things contain aspects of both and it would probably be better to talk about a continuum. A bed-sore, for instance, has physical reality, but is also socially constructed in a certain sense. However, if our research is centrally concerned with the sore and not with its multiple cultural meanings, we may be methodologically justified in bracketing the social for the time being. It is important to remember that methodological reductionism is not problematic in the same way as 'real' ontological reductionism.

One may wonder why qualitative researchers are so interested in (or obsessed with?) philosophy since most qualitative research projects and methodologies can be accommodated within standard philosophy of science without any major problems. The specific methodological precepts in quantitative research are often antithetical to the methodological precepts of qualitative research, but at the deeper level of underlying philosophy of science there is no necessary conflict. One way of bringing about this *rapprochement* is through the pragmatist philosopher C.S. Peirce and his analysis of abduction (or 'inference to best explanation') as a valid mode of inference alongside deduction and induction (Peirce, 1878 and 1898; Lipton, 1991). By a close analysis of the inferential steps in a number of qualitative methodologies it is possible to show that they employ abduction in the final steps of the analysis, as well as deduction and induction in the intermediate steps (Holm, 1997). The same can be shown for quantitative research, where abductive inferences abound in the typical research papers 'discussion' section. The large surface differences between qualitative and quantitative methodologies are thus misleading. They hide a fundamental similarity in inferential procedure. It is therefore possible to evaluate and assess qualitative methodologies and the results from qualitative studies in a way that is just as rigorous as our evaluation of quantitative results and methods.

Let's go continental!

One of the possibilities for a separate philosophical foundation for qualitative research is some form of so-called 'continental' philosophy, like phenomenology, hermeneutics, or Habermasian critical social research (Gadamer, 1990; Habermas, 1990). It is therefore of interest to analyse whether a qualitative approach built on such a different philosophical foundation would necessarily fall outside the EBP framework.

The first thing to note is that 'continental' philosophy is not one monolithic school of philosophy, but an artificial bundling together of some very, very different philosophers whose only common feature is that they do not belong to the school of Anglo-American analytic philosophy. There is, therefore, very little that, for instance, connects Habermas and Heidegger at the level of basic philosophy.

Due to space constraints and lack of the appropriate philosophical expertise I am not going to look at all of the different 'continental' philosophies, but will confine myself to phenomenology, which is generally recognized as the foundation of an important phenomenological school of qualitative researchers (Schutz, 1962; Giorgi, 1985; Moustakas, 1994; Creswell, 1998)[8]. The German philosopher Edmund Husserl was the founder of phenomenology. His work was expanded and in that process changed by later phenomenologists like Martin Heidegger in Germany and Maurice Merleau-Ponty in France Husserl, 1950; Merleau-Ponty, 1962; Hammond *et al.*, 1991; Heidegger, 1993).

Part of Husserl's philosophical project was a fundamental opposition to the prevalent positivism of his day, but it is important to note that he wanted to supplant it with a new form of science that was just as methodologically rigorous and scientifically precise as its positivistic predecessor (Kolakowski, 1987). Husserl criticized the naïve view that we have direct access to the external world and that perception is an essentially passive enterprise. He pointed out that perception is always intentional, in that it is directed at something.

Intentionality, or the sense in which something is *directed towards* its object, is seen by phenomenologists as a characteristic and basic constituent of every conscious mental phenomenon, and of every conscious act. All conscious acts are directed towards something. Our very consciousness projects itself towards the world around us. When we perceive something our consciousness is itself always already part of what we perceive: the object of our perception is not given to us directly, but is partly constituted by an active, directed *act* of perception.[9]

However, phenomenologists are not necessarily *phenomenalist*, that is, they do not think that our world is essentially one of experiences or sensations rather than real objects external to us (nor do they claim, with Kant, that we have access only to a mentally constructed world rather than to hidden, underlying objects). For Husserl, perception of phenomena is caused by the world, and the purpose of the phenomenological analysis (usually called 'the phenomenological reduction' in the phenomenological literature) is to discover the invariant features of a given percept in order to gain knowledge about the world (Hintikka, 1995). He further believed that we are able to get secure knowledge since some perceptions give themselves to us as self-evidently (apodictically) certain, meaning that they cannot be doubted. This latter point on the self-evidence of certain perceptions has been criticized from many sides (Kolakowski, 1987), but the phenomenological project of reducing our experiences to what is self-given does not stand or fall with the existence of self-evident perceptions.

In describing the epistemology of the phenomenologists – that is, their understanding of what knowledge is, and of how knowledge is available to us – it is important to emphasize that one of the aims is to give a better account of everyday experiences and not simply to form a secure basis for scientific knowledge. The concepts of 'lived-experience' and 'lived-world' therefore become central in many phenomenological analyses of aspects of human life.

In his early works Heidegger critically extended Husserl's epistemological ideas by pointing out that our primary access to the world and the things in it is not primarily through an analytic gaze or perception of the phenomena, but through relations of use with equipment (*Zeug*) that is ready to hand (*Zuhande*). Thus I learn most about a hammer not by looking at it or theorizing about it, but by using it for hammering. In Heidegger's own words in *Being and Time*:

> Equipment can genuinely show itself only in dealings cut to its own measure (hammering with a hammer, for example); but in such dealings an entity of this kind is not *grasped* thematically as an occurring Thing, nor is the equipment-structure known as such in the using... the less we just stare at the hammer-thing, and the more we seize hold of it and use it, the more primordial does our relationship to it become, and the more unveiledly is it encountered as that which it is – as equipment. The hammering itself uncovers the specific 'manipulability' of the hammer. The kind of Being which equipment possesses – in which it manifests itself in it own right – we call '*readiness-to-hand*'. Only because equipment has *this* 'Being-in-itself' and does not merely occur, is it manipulable in the broadest sense and at our disposal. No matter how sharply we just *look* at the 'outward appearance' of Things in whatever form this takes, we cannot discover anything ready-to-hand. If we look at Things just 'theoretically', we can get along without understanding readiness-to-hand. (Heidegger, 1962, p. 98, emphasis in original)

Merleau-Ponty extended the epistemology of Husserl in a different direction by pointing to the importance of the body for my understanding of myself and my world. Just like I have a 'lived world', I also am a 'lived body'. He argued that the Cartesian dualism between mind and body has to be overcome through a realization that I do not *have* a body; I *am* a body. A true phenomenology of the human condition must take this into account. Every perception necessarily involves the body in a non-trivial sense. Or as Merleau-Ponty himself writes:

> Our bodily experience of movement is not a particular case of knowledge; it provides us with a way of access to the world and the object, with a 'praktognosia', which has to be recognised as original and perhaps as primary. My body has its world, or understands its world, without having to make use of my 'symbolic' or 'objectifying function'. (Merleau-Ponty, 1962, pp. 140–141)

It should be evident from the above that phenomenological philosophy differs in many ways from Anglo-American analytic philosophy. The important question in the present context is, however, whether the differences in epistemology would make the EBP enterprise invalid within a phenomenological frame. The answer to this question is, perhaps surprisingly, 'No'. Although phenomenologists have quite specific views about what sorts of knowledge we can acquire, how we gain knowledge, as well as what the limits for our knowledge are, they would have no problems with the basic tenets of the EBP enterprise. They would all quite happily subscribe to the view that I can only act appropriately in the world if I possess valid knowledge about it. They would claim that the knowledge that 'science' gives is not the most fundamental level of knowledge, but they would not reject it. That there is more to be known does not mean that what I already know becomes invalid. A phenomenologist and an EBP practitioner would probably have great initial communication problems, but they would in the end be able to speak to each other.

The dangers of second-hand knowledge

Mastering qualitative research methodologies at a level enabling one to perform independent research is a time-consuming enterprise. The move from novice to expert takes many years for most of us. But we have been told either explicitly, or implicitly from the composition of the extant literature, that we also have to be able to defend qualitative research (or at least our own particular approach) on the philosophical level. In the introduction to one of the standard handbooks on qualitative research methodology advocating the role as *bricoleur* for the researcher, we read for instance:

> The *bricoleur* is adept at performing a large number of diverse tasks, ranging from interviewing to observing, to interpreting personal and historical documents, to intensive self-reflection and introspection. The *bricoleur* reads widely and is knowledgeable about the many interpretive paradigms (feminism, Marxism, cultural studies, constructivism) that can be brought to any particular problem. He or she may not, however, feel that paradigms can be mingled, or synthesized. That is, paradigms as overarching philosophical systems denoting particular ontologies, epistemologies, and methodologies cannot easily be moved between. They represent belief systems that attach the user to a particular worldview. (Denzin and Lincoln, 1998, p. 4)

To gain the amount of knowledge required here is obviously a tall order, even if we do not take account of the standard Kuhnian insight that a paradigm cannot be fully explicated if you are working within it and cannot be fully understandable if you are looking at it from the outside. Going to the primary literature (that is, the literature of the relevant philosophers) is both time-consuming and difficult for the philosophically untrained. There is, therefore, a temptation to learn the philosophy underlying the chosen method from secondary literature such as short introductions to the philosopher(s) or, even worse, from tertiary literature such as presentations of the philosopher(s)' writings by qualitative methodologists who rely on secondary literature, and to quote this secondary or tertiary literature in one's own writing as if it accurately reflected the position of the philosopher(s) in question.[10]

This is, however, extremely dangerous and may border on the academically dishonest. The secondary writers may not truly have understood the philosophy they are writing about,[11] and even if they have, paraphrasing often hides important ambiguities and subtleties. If, as an example, we look at a philosopher like the phenomenologist Martin Heidegger,[12] there is general agreement that his works are written in an extremely difficult German and that his position and his use of central concepts change on crucial points during his life (Steiner, 1992; Guignon, 1993). The collected edition of his works is still in publication and there are a planned 65 volumes of writings and 35 additional volumes of comments, letters, fragments and such-like. Most of these writings have never been translated into English. Among Heidegger scholars it is acknowledged that he is at times almost untranslatable, and that the standard translations of some of his major works to English are deficient in various ways.[13] In secondary writing on Heidegger in English, authors often prefer to modify the standard translation of the sections they quote. If we confine ourselves to Heidegger's epistemology, it turns out that the early Heidegger has different views from the late Heidegger on many important issues, including the proper analysis of knowledge claims and the correct analysis of truth. The primacy of knowledge through the use of equipment (*Zeug*) that is ready to hand (*Zuhande*) over the mere perception of items that are present at hand (*Vorhanden*) is, for instance, a view that is prominent in Heidegger's early work *Being and Time* but disappears in his later writings (Tugendhat, 1967; Heidegger, 1993).

Knowing and referring to the views of Heidegger is thus not a simple matter, and there is a significant risk that what one is referring to is not Heidegger, but the pseudo-Heidegger constructed by some secondary source. It has been argued that both Heidegger and Husserl have mainly been misunderstood by nursing researchers (Paley, 1997 and 1998). In an EBP context it could also be argued that long excurses into philosophy (or pseudo-philosophy) are unlikely to alter the final value of a research project, which stands or falls not with Heidegger or some other philosopher, but with the soundness of the methodology and its competent execution.

Conclusion

In this chapter it has been argued that qualitative research is not excluded from the EBP framework but a necessary part of it. It has been argued further that the discussion about different paradigms for quantitative and qualitative research and the rejection of EBP because of its affiliation with the quantitative paradigm is misguided (unless one adopts a strong social constructivist position). The EBP framework is not incompatible with the philosophy underlying qualitative research, and the EBP requirements for quality in research are as easily met by qualitative as by quantitative researchers.

Notes

1. In this chapter I use the term 'intervention' to cover all forms of direct medical and surgical treatments and diagnostic interventions,

all caring interventions, and all the different ways of organizing treatment and care which have an influence on the patient's experiences in the health care environment (a specific way of organizing nursing care in a department would thus be an intervention for the purposes of this chapter).

2. I am here using 'paradigm shift' in a fairly loose sense. It can be argued that before 1850 medicine was still in the pre-scientific stage and that no dominant paradigm in a Kuhnian sense had yet been established.

3. Epistemology is the part of philosophy which deals with the justification of knowledge claims. According to the classic definition, knowledge is true, justified belief. A knowledge claim's epistemic warrant is the sum total of the reasons I can give for believing it to be true.

4. Uncontroversial seen from the point of view of EBP. Relegating qualitative research to the role of a pilot before 'real' research is obviously controversial and problematic seen from the point of view of the qualitative researcher.

5. For the record I find the qualitative/quantitative distinction less then helpful and would instead prefer to talk about interpretative and non-interpretative research (Holm, 1997), but in deference to the standard usage I will use qualitative and quantitative here.

6. Far from all health interventions aim at changing hard endpoints like death, infection rates or length of stay in hospital.

7. In some recent social constructivist writings 'we' have also moved beyond post-positivism (Guba and Lincoln, 1998), although the historical account of post-positivism which is given by Guba and Lincoln is woefully deficient.

8. The following brief exposition of phenomenology does not claim to be a sufficient basis for a full understanding of this school of philosophy. It should especially be noted that it does not give a fully adequate account of the philosophical differences between the phenomenologists mentioned.

9. The pleonastic nature of the phrase 'active act' is unavoidable when we consider Husserl's ideas of perception, for whom perception was an *act* in the sense of being undertaken by an agent, and *active* in the sense of engaged with its object, whether consciously or not.

10. An example of this problematic practice can be found in the paper from which the quote above is taken (Denzin and Lincoln, 1998), where the only reference the authors give for the ontology of the positivist and post-positivist paradigms is Guba (1990), which is not a primary reference to a positivist or post-positivist philosopher or research methodologist, but a secondary reference to an opponent of positivism and post-positivism.

11. This is especially a problem if one gains the knowledge from reading the works of the opponents of a particular position.

12. There is even disagreement whether (the early) Heidegger should be classified as a phenomenologist or as an existentialist. Jean-Paul Sartre saw him as an existentialist forerunner in his *Being and Nothingness*.

13. This is for instance the case for his major early work *Sein und Zeit*, where the two extant translations differ significantly in places (Heidegger, 1993, 1962 and 1996).

References

In order to ease further study, most references to non-English authors are to available translations. As mentioned above, sole reliance on translation may, however, be problematic in some cases.

Bowling, A. (1997) *Measuring health: a review of quality of life measurement scales*, 2nd edn, Buckingham: Open University Press.

Burke, K. (1999) 'NICE and easy', *Nursing Standard*, **13** (30): 13.

Collin, F. (1997) *Social Reality*, London: Routledge.

Creswell, J.W. (1998) *Qualitative Inquiry and Research Design: Choosing Among Five Traditions*, Thousand Oaks, CA: Sage Publications.

Denzin, N.K. and Lincoln, Y.S. (1998) 'Introduction – Entering the Field of Qualitative Research', in Denzin, N.K. and Lincoln, Y.S. (eds) *The Landscape of Qualitative Research: Theories and Issues*, Thousand Oaks, CA: Sage Publications.

Evidence-based medicine working group (1992) 'Evidence-based medicine: a new approach to teaching the practice of medicine', *JAMA*, **268**: 2420–2425.

Feinstein, A.R. and Horwitz, R.I. (1997) 'Problems in the "Evidence" of "Evidence-based Medicine"', *American Journal of Medicine*, **103** (6): 529–535.

Gadamer, H.-G. (1990) *Wahrheit und Methode: Grundzüge einer Philosophischen Hermeneutik* (6. Aufl.), Tübingen: J.C.B. Mohr.

Gergen, K.J. and Gergen, M.M. (1991) 'Toward reflexive methodologies', in Steier, F. (ed.) *Research and Reflexivity*, London: Sage Publications.

Giorgi, A. (ed.) (1985) *Phenomenology and psychological research*, Pittsburgh, PA: Duquesne University Press.

Griffin, J. (1986) *Well-being: its meaning, measurement and moral importance*, Oxford: Clarendon.

Guba, E.G. (1990) 'The alternative paradigm dialog', in Guba, E.G. (ed.) *The paradigm dialog*, Newbury Park, CA: Sage Publications.

Guba, E.G. and Lincoln, Y.S. (1998) 'Competing Paradigms in Qualitative Research', in Denzin, N.K. and Lincoln, Y.S. (eds) *The Landscape of Qualitative Research: Theories and Issues*, Thousand Oaks, CA: Sage Publications.

Guignon, C. (ed.) (1993) *The Cambridge Companion to Heidegger*, Cambridge: Cambridge University Press.

Habermas, J. (1990) *Moral Consciousness and Communicative Action*, Cambridge, MA: Polity Press.

Hammond, M., Howarth, J. and Keat, R. (1991) *Understanding Phenomenology*, Oxford: Blackwell Publishers.

Heidegger, M. (1962) *Being and Time*, trans. J. Macqarrie & E. Robinson, London: Blackwell Publishers.

Heidegger, M. (1993) *Sein und Zeit* (17. Aufl.), Tübingen: Max Niemeyer Verlag.

Heidegger, M. (1996) *Being and Time*, trans. J. Stambaugh, Albany: SUNY Press.

Hintikka, J. (1995) 'The Phenomenological Dimension', in Smith, B. and Smith, D.W. (eds) *The Cambridge Companion to Husserl*, Cambridge: Cambridge University Press.

Holm, S. (1997) *Ethical problems in clinical practice: The ethical reasoning of health care professionals*, Manchester: Manchester University Press.

Husserl, E. (1950) *Cartesian Meditations – An Introduction to Phenomenology*, The Hague: Martinus Nijhoff.

Kolakowski, L. (1987) *Husserl and the Search for Certitude*, Chicago, IL: Chicago University Press.

Kvale, S. (1989) *Issues of Validity in Qualitative Research*, Lund: Studentlitteratur.

Lipton, P. (1991) *Inference to the Best Explanation*, London: Routledge.

Merleau-Ponty, M. (1962) *Phenomenology of Perception*, London: Routledge and Kegan Paul.

Morse, J.M. (ed.) (1994) *Critical Issues in Qualitative Research Methodologies*, Thousand Oaks, CA: Sage Publications.

Moustakas, C. (1994) *Phenomenological research methods*, Thousand Oaks, CA: Sage Publications.

O'Reilly, M. (1997) 'Evidence-based medicine designed to save physicians time, energy, FPs told', *CMAJ*, **156** (10): 1457–1458.

Paley, J. (1997) 'Husserl, phenomenology and nursing', *Journal of Advanced Nursing*, **26** (1): 187–193.

Paley, J. (1998) 'Misinterpretive phenomenology: Heidegger, ontology and nursing research', *Journal of Advanced Nursing*, **27** (4): 817–824.

Peirce, C.S. (1878 [1992]) 'Deduction, induction, and hypothesis', in Houser, N. and Kloesel, C. (eds) *The Essential Peirce – Selected Philosophical Writings* (Vol. 1), Bloomington, IN: Indiana University Press.

Peirce, C.S. (1898 [1992]) 'Reasoning and the logic of things', in Ketner, K.L. (ed.) *Reasoning and the Logic of Things – Charles Sanders Peirce*, Cambridge, MA: Harvard University Press.

Polkinghorne, D.E. (1983) *Methodology for the Human Sciences*, Albany, NY: SUNY Press.

Porter, S. (1996) 'Qualitative Analysis', in Cormack, D.F.S. (ed.) *The Research Process in Nursing*, 3rd edn, Oxford: Blackwell Science.

Sackett, D.L., Rosenberg, W.M.C., Muir Gray, J.A. *et al.* (1996) 'Evidence based medicine: what it is and what it isn't', *BMJ*, **312**: 71–72.

Sackett, D.L., Straus, S.E., Richardson, W.S. *et al.* (2000) *Evidence-Based Medicine: How to Practice and Teach EBM*, London: Churchill Livingstone.

Schutz, A. (1962) *Collected Papers: The Problem of Social Reality*, The Hague: Martinus Nijhoff Publishers.

Steiner, G. (1992) *Heidegger*, 2nd edn, London: Fontana Press.

Tugendhat, E. (1967) *Der Wahrheitsbegriff bei Husserl und Heidegger*, Berlin: Walter de Gruyter.

Upton, D. (1999) 'How can we achieve evidence-based practice if we have a theory-practice gap in nursing today?' *Journal of Advanced Nursing*, **29** (3): 549–555.

4

Nursing's Role in Shaping European Health Policy

Tom Keighley

Introduction

The notion of Europe is both old and new. Its current construction flows directly from the decisions taken in the aftermath of the Second World War. This comparative recency of creation is a major influence when considering policy formulation. Significant differences in approaches to decision-making, goal-setting and outcome evaluation have yet to be resolved even within structured organizations like the European Union (EU). Achieving unity of approach, let alone consistency of delivery, is still a struggle. Europe is an emergent political framework, constantly changing, as new groupings are developed and new alliances agreed.

To consider health care, let alone nursing, in such a situation is a challenge. The notion of 'health' itself varies greatly across the continent, as do the systems that provide health care. The roles of individual professions and public expectations about their performance also vary. This goes beyond assessing the balance of health care delivery by comparing the extent of primary care provision in contrast to hospital services. It strikes at the fundamental value placed on health care and the role of non-medical staff, especially the status of women as providers of care in both formal and informal settings.

Determining the role of nursing in shaping health policy is therefore difficult. While it is possible to point to some significant achievements, the national variations in the structure of the nurse's role and the nursing profession, the degree of integration into national policy formulation and the educational level achieved at first registration seem to be key determinants. Underpinning all efforts to influence health policy is the level of preparedness that nurse leaders have reached, in particular, to what degree political skills have been developed. Above all else, influencing the development of health policy in Europe depends on the resources available and the long-term commitment to pursue goals.

Summary

To put the above into the current context for nursing in Europe, this chapter provides some historical background and an initial focus on the principal areas of pan-European cooperation in relation to both the nursing profession's influence on health policy and professional education. An assessment of the stage of development of nursing practice, nursing management and nursing research as policy influencers is then provided. The chapter concludes with a view about the future and some suggestions about involvement in lobbying.

Background

In some respects, what is being resolved in Europe today is the consequence of Christmas Day, AD 800. On that day, Charlemagne was crowned Holy Roman Emperor in a vain attempt by the Pope and the residual powers of a rapidly crumbling state to maintain stability and provide structure to a land mass threatened by invasion from the north and the east. It was a political move based on the hypothesis that there was a grouping of countries that had benefited from the administrative and trade links that the western Roman Empire had created and were now bound together by a common religion. Whether they saw it as a Commonwealth of Nations or a rudimentary common market is unclear. What it did was to legitimate the Carolingian monarchy in its right to rule outside of its original Frankish domain, and so began the process of creating a political entity that has come to be known as Europe.

The spread of the Byzantine Empire northwest into what is now known as the former Russian Empire brought a different set of expectations about unifying nations but with an essentially Romanesque bias. As a result, from the tenth century onwards, a land mass that stretched from the Ural Mountains to the Summer Isles off Galway, and the Mediterranean littoral to Scandinavia, was perceived as representing an interrelated group of nations and peoples. The politics of this has led to a millennium of political struggle, which has too often spilled over on to battlefields. The fallout from the greatest of these political breakdowns led to the creation of the Europe of today. Even here, however, it is important to note that the boundaries are not fixed, as nations in the former countries of Eastern Europe struggle to establish themselves. Nearer to home, peoples within the larger geographic groupings are pressing with vigour for greater independence. This was apparent in the UK when considering the devolution of Scotland and Wales and in the degree of independence that the federated states of Germany or Spain are exercising. The internal boundaries of Europe are fluid when considered in the medium term.

Nursing in Europe

The history of nursing in Europe varies significantly across the continent. Probably the only common factor is the influence of the Christian faith in all its many traditions. Many countries date the modern era of nursing from the point at which they implemented their own version of the Nightingale reforms. Nightingale herself, however, trained under the guidance of a Lutheran community at Kaiserwerth. Her regard for the other major nursing tradition in Europe, the Sisters of Charity, led her, at the start of the Crimean War, to try to attract some of the English-speaking Sisters from the community in Paris to join her (Woodham-Smith, 1950, pp. 89–91 and 147).

The pre-existence of such structured nursing resources on the European mainland is important when considering the ability of nurses to influence health policy. The Nightingale tradition with its strong roots in Protestantism has always encompassed a political element. In contrast, the Roman Catholic tradition had not developed at the time of Nightingale and, in many respects, still struggles to develop the overt political tendencies of other nursing traditions. It is possible to posit a European north/south divide in this respect. Such analysis of divides is only useful as a reflective tool to illuminate national and supranational differences. Other comparisons would be the comparative proportion of doctors to nurses, the number of hospital beds to community care staff, or the provision of specialist medical care in comparison with primary health care as highlighted in Chapter 2. The degree of variation in these factors highlights the variation that has emerged within the different nursing workforces in Europe.

After 1945, it was apparent that the initial contacts that had begun to emerge before the war between the different nurse associations should be reawakened despite the differences in national position and professional structure. The detailed story of this is recounted by Quinn and Russell (1993, pp. 13–14). By the late 1960s, two influential pieces of work were under way. The first was the establishment of the Standing Committee of Nursing (known as PCN from the French translation), which was finally completed in 1971. The second was the initial work on draft directives for the general nursing part of the profession by the European Commission. Both of these initiatives owed much to the work of the staff of the International Council of Nurses (ICN), who during the 1950s facilitated and chaired many of the meetings that enabled the passage of change.

European directives on the nurse responsible for general care

The development, implementation and subsequent history of these directives make an illustrative case history of the ability of the profession to influence policy in Europe. There is the implicit assumption in this statement that the principal organization to influence is the European Union. This is true in so far as EU law supersedes national law, meaning that unless derogation (a technical term for an exemption) has been sought, national governments must implement EU agreements. It is therefore the organization with greatest power.

In the initial discussions following the signing of the Treaty of Rome in 1957, draft directives for the professions were drawn up. The purpose of these was to ensure free movement of personnel between member countries based on the principle of mutual recognition. This mutual recognition was to be based on the commonality of training content, both theoretical and practical. The predecessor of the PCN, the Western European Nursing Group (GNOE, again from the French) had commenced negotiations with the ECC (European Communities [predecessor of the EU] Commission) in 1961. The discussions took on new momentum with a report issued by a working party of the

Council of Europe in 1967. This organization had been established at intergovernmental level immediately after the war to ensure a forum existed for governments from across the whole of Europe to meet and determine joint policy. The signing of an Agreement on Nurse Training (Council of Europe, 1967) by the member states of the Council of Europe brought things to a head and the EEC submitted draft directives to the European Parliament for comment in 1970.

Despite having reached this stage of development, it was 1975 before the EC Council of Ministers convened an intergovernmental group of experts to agree the final content of the directives. What followed was one of the key discussions between the then ECC and the profession. The sticking point was on duration of training. The Commission was proposing 3,700 hours while members of the Council of Europe had already signed up to 4,600 hours. Subsequent discussion saw the Commission shift its position. In 1977 the directives on the training and activities of the general nurse became ECC law, along with two decisions by the Council of Ministers on the establishment of the Advisory Committee on the Training of Nurses (ACTN), and the division between theory and practice. This was the product of a concerted piece of lobbying, led by the PCN and the National Nurse Associations (NNAs).

These directives are still the foundation of the profession's relationship with the EU and its Commission, although this may be set to change. Similar directives were passed for midwifery, medicine and dentistry in the health care field. These directives establish a competency (a technical term meaning legitimate authority) in the EU to take a formal interest in nursing. The development brought together two points of influence: the PCN as the official liaison committee for the Commission on all issues relating to nursing, and the ACTN as an instrument in law which had to be consulted by the Commission on all issues specific to nurse training. Over time a shared membership between the two committees has occurred in the representation of some countries. This, along with increasingly effective patterns of communication, has ensured that the profession has become influential in Brussels and therefore in much of western Europe.

The Commission is currently revising legislation in relation to all professional qualifications (EU, COM (2002) 119 Final) including nurses, midwives and doctors and a consultation exercise on an EU proposal is currently under way. Once approved, all the Advisory Committees, including that for the training of nurses, will be disbanded; meetings of the ACTN are currently suspended.

Europe and nurse education

From the description of the work done on nurse education, it is clear that this has been the main unifying feature of nursing's efforts to influence policy formulation in the health care arena. This is probably because there was material evidence on which to work. It is very difficult to establish what is standard practice in any area of nursing care within a country, let alone to get agreement on how to change and develop it at international level. However, in education, the existence of curricula and regulatory bodies to overview their use and application gives a concrete base for discussion and joint development. The recognition of this common ground goes hand in glove with the needs of the principal political force in Europe, that is, the EU, to pursue a separate agenda on the free movement of labour. It is seren-dipitous that the two agendas have come together.

The profession has not handled even the nurse education agenda as a unified whole. This is evidenced by the activities of the Council of Europe and the World Health Organization (WHO) Europe. Mention has already been made of the Council of Europe report in 1967. In 1994, a further report was issued (Council of Europe, 1994). This was a timely, if unplanned, contribution to a debate within the ACTN on the reform of the general nurse directives. However, it is still difficult to trace the policy motivation within the Council of Europe that led to this work being commissioned.

Another example of this was the work undertaken by WHO Europe in 1988. As a result of a WHO conference held in Vienna in that year, a decision was reached to pursue the development of the generic nurse (WHO, 1989). This has proved to be a fundamental threat to the maintenance of the pre-registration specialist education programmes in mental health, learning disabilities and paediatric nursing. It is not such an issue on the European mainland, where many countries do not have such specialist preparation at either pre- or post-registration levels. However, it has placed a divide between those countries that require the education of such nurses in their health care systems and those that do not. Currently, WHO Europe has undertaken another review of nurse education with the intention of offering further guid-ance to the profession to reflect the future direction of health care needs emerging from the WHO development of its policy on *Health For All in the Twenty-First Century* (WHO, 1998). This was issued in 2000 (WHO, 2000). These examples demonstrate well the complexity of influencing nursing education policy in Europe.

The key issue concerns the legitimate remit of different organizations and what their current agendas might be. Added to this is the need to recognize who and what is driving the agenda and what the political aims might be. The three organizations that have been considered so far are all driven by the requirements of their constituency. In each case it is the member governments that set the agenda and fund the work. This means that the officers of those organizations are constrained by the supranational framework within which they work. This is not to suggest that the officers are unable to influence the agenda, only that they have very little leeway in the initiation of work or the utilization of resources. This is often useful to the member governments, who can use these organizations as the scapegoats for the implementation of nationally unpopular policies. This position of dependence makes the implementation of policies from these organizations particularly susceptible to delay and prevarication.

A major concern has been the development of specialist nurse education in the EU. The ACTN has been involved in the development of education in the fields of cancer (CEC, 1988) and in the care of elderly people (CEC, 1994). These have provided insight into the development of specialist nursing in the EU and have led to a series of reviews conducted by the committee on how specialist nursing is developing. It is of concern to the EC because such developments may lead to restraints on the free movement of labour. The picture that is emerging is of increasing provision of post-basic specialist education, nearly always based in higher education. This is critical because it points to a European-wide shift of nurse education away from local technical schools and hospital-based facilities towards a research-based culture.

This is not a universally agreed development across the EU, and some countries are working to obstruct the move. However, as health care provision becomes more specialist and the costs of health care delivery rise, external pressures are leading to the implementation of this change, as Evers highlights in Chapter 2. Limiting the speed of change are two important factors: the status of nursing as a profession, and the value placed on caring in the different EU countries. The presence of strong NNAs has facilitated the change and, in countries where they are absent, has led to only slow progress. Other difficulties include the lack of senior specialist nurses to teach the subjects, and no recognition system to enable the education to be used elsewhere when nurses change jobs.

Against this background the PCN has convened meetings to learn from the extant specialist nurse groups in Europe how to develop a joint approach to this issue. The EC has commissioned a legal study of the development of specialist nurse education to consider the nature of the current provision at both pre- and post-registration levels. This will be helpful because it will identify any problems not covered by the current directives arising from recognition of qualifications in other countries, and why politicians and doctors in some countries are so resistant to the development.

The focus on the education of nurses is also heavily influenced by the developing public health agenda in Europe. While many observers may see this as being led by WHO, the contribution of the EU in this field of activity has expanded dramatically since the Maastricht Treaty (1992), when the EC was formally granted competence in this area of work and has been further developed within the Amsterdam Treaty (1998). The implications for nursing from the work of the WHO and the EU in the field of public health are significant. It confirms the shift in health care towards primary care and emphasizes disease prevention as much as hospital-based care for the sick. This shift in part explains the need to reflect on the nature of nursing education. However, even more significant are the demographic changes within Europe. Drawing on the EUROSTAT data, Ludvigsen and Roberts (1996, p. 93) paint a picture of ever-increasing numbers of older people and a diminishing workforce to both care for them and to fund their care through taxes or insurance.

Looking forward twenty years or so, this projects a scenario where nurses and nursing services will be in high demand. Also the users of health care services will be better informed about the options facing them as the impact of the information revolution together with resource constraints will have increased public concern about the effectiveness and efficiency of the therapies offered. Nurses will need to be sufficiently educated to both negotiate the delivery of care and to be able to assure service users that they are providing the pattern of care most recommended for the particular problem. Also, many people will want access to nurses to help interpret the lifestyle information they will have gleaned from the mass of electronic media in their homes. It is a future that offers many opportunities for the development of the nursing profession and is also one that hinges on access to appropriate levels of higher education.

Europe and nursing practice

It is difficult to assess the impact of nursing practice on policy formulation in Europe. While nurse education emerges from and in turn influences the nature of nursing practice, there has been little by way of assessment of nursing practice in the form of cross-national comparisons and surveys. As a result, there is a marked variation in expectations about nursing practice both between countries and in many instances within a single country. This is especially true where the provinces or regions of a particular country have high levels of autonomy in their decision-making. However, some landmark developments have occurred.

One significant event was the emergence of the European Oncology Nursing Society (EONS). While not the first of the pan-European nursing groups, it was the first to successfully tag a development in the EC. Following the declaration of the 'War on Cancer' in the 1980s, the EC put large amounts of money into research and development in this area. The result was that EONS made a number of bids to attract that money to help it establish a European-wide organization, a journal and training programmes at various centres in different parts of Europe. This led to the production of a core curriculum to ensure achievement of a common standard. This activity also attracted money from other sources. As a result, the organization has become a powerful lobby in its own right. A key element of this was its ability to work with doctors in pursuit of a common aim.

Another organization that has established a powerful European presence is the Federation of Occupational Health Nurses within the EU (FOHNEU). Its motivation was to try to influence the development and implementation of legislation to effect the health and welfare of people at work. Many of the nurses in this group work for organizations whose corporate policies take a European if not a global approach to business. In contrast to the more clinically based approach of EONS, FOHNEU has lobbied national and EU politicians, as well as the most senior members of the Commission. It exemplifies an approach based on sound professional knowledge and a wish to be active in the political arena.

These two examples are taken from perhaps twenty such nursing groups active across Europe whose interests range from the exchange of information about professional practice through more academic interests to those that are overtly political. The challenge facing the profession is how to align the interests of these specialist groups to the broader-based interests of the NNAs. Studying the nature of the education of such specialists is one way into this issue. Another, and one that is perhaps more important, is to consider how the overt interest that they have in professional practice and patient care can be brought to bear on the social dialogue of the EU, which too often is tied to the terms and conditions of employment. Equally there are concerns that the apparently ever-burgeoning specialist groups will lead to a splintering of the NNAs, resulting in a loss of their current base for policy formulation and international influence. It is a development that is beginning to unsettle those NNAs that have not managed to retain the specialist nursing groups among their membership.

Europe, nursing research and leadership

In terms of formation, these groups could be described as the oldest and the newest 'kids on the block'. The Workgroup of European Nurse Researchers (WENR) was established in the late 1970s as the nursing process swept through Europe. In contrast the nurse managers or, as they are known in the different countries of Europe, administrators, have only recently formed an organization and are still formulating their way of working. However, both groups share the same difficulty within Europe, that of recognition. This is because there is no easy way of establishing the political relevance of their contribution. There is no doubt about the value placed on the individuals concerned by both their organizations and their colleagues.

It was almost impossible for nurse researchers to win research monies in their own right from the EU until the changes introduced in the Fifth Framework (the title for the research disbursement scheme in the EU) improved nursing's opportunities. Within this framework, a number of nursing research projects have been successful in their bids for EU funding. As nursing has developed as an academic subject in Europe, the various members of WENR have provided support at both personal and individual levels. As a consequence, nursing research has risen higher on the national agendas, a prerequisite for its successful management on the international agenda.

Senior nurses often hold an ambivalent place in NNAs, especially when the NNA is also a trade union. This is because senior nurses often appear on the management side in any dispute. As a result, nurses have become involved in a number of the multidisciplinary management groups, and in the emergence of a specific European group to enable nurse leadership to appear on political agendas in its own right through the WHO Europe office. The regular convening of meetings, by WHO Europe, of Chief Nurses in Government, has supported this development. The progression of the autonomous hospital movement across Europe, typified by the creation of NHS Trusts in the UK, is also giving a degree of prominence to nurse leadership that was previously lacking. This is an emerging agenda at a European level.

The future

The development of the WHO policy, *Health for All in the Twenty-First Century*, will have a continuing impact on health care policy formulation across Europe and will help determine the nature of both nurse education and nursing practice, especially as the shift to primary care accelerates. As the European public health agenda unfolds, it will also reflect Article 152 of the Amsterdam Treaty, with its emphasis on:

- Health protection in policy formulation
- The development of public health
- Renewed focus on the management of communicable diseases
- New initiatives on major disease challenges, for instance, substance misuse.

This range of work will be heavily influenced by the other major change in the health and economic status of the EU, namely the admission of new countries, including: Bulgaria, Cyprus, the Czech Republic, Estonia, Hungary, Latvia, Lithuania, Malta, Poland, Romania, Slovakia and Slovenia. Many of these countries have not developed their health care staff or systems in a way that is comparable to, or compatible with, the EU. Added to this, they have a range and depth of public health problems arising from their environmental management that will take many decades to resolve (Saltman and Figueras,

1997, pp. 15–24). The Commission already realizes that a more coordinated approach to health is required. Currently, while the Maastricht and Amsterdam Treaties health agenda is being managed within Directorate General (DG) for Health and Consumer Protection, at least ten other DGs have health-related responsibilities, including those responsible for:

- Enlargement
- Enterprise and Information Society
- Agriculture, Rural development and Fisheries
- Transport and Energy
- Environment
- Justice and Social Affairs
- Research.

This disjunction can result in fragmentation, as there is no require-ment to consult in the development of policy. Walter Mathias for the European Health Care Managers' Association (EHMA) has reviewed this lack of cohesion in health care policy development in an unpub-lished study. He has identified 97 directives that relate to health care, a third of which have emerged from the European Court as a result of citizens challenging the interpretation of various EU agreements. In reality, therefore, a framework for health care in the EU has come into existence. It has arisen because politicians have not appreciated the implications of the agreements they have signed. Many of the directives make no mention of health care but because they have established general principles, it is as these are applied to health care that their significance in this area emerges.

The combination, therefore, of a new competence in health care awarded to the Commission, a joint agenda on public health by both the WHO and the EU, and the admission of several new member states in the next five years will change the approach to health care delivery significantly. Added to this are the demographic changes referred to earlier. This all suggests a significant role extension for the nurse, especially as increasing amounts of health care will be delivered at home. The need for higher education for nurses becomes apparent in this scenario, and related to this, an increasing number of nurses in all countries will need to be equipped to contrib-ute to the research and analysis of these changes and the responses to them.

Lobbying

The need to influence the formation of European health policy means that the profession must develop and work through various networks. Mention has already been made of the evolution of the PCN and the joint working of the NNAs to influence the thinking of the EU. This has been developed into the establishment of a permanent, full-time lobby function in Brussels on behalf of the PCN. The NNAs work through this as well as through their individual lobby resources to acquire information about the emerging agenda and to identify opportunities for consultation and negotiation. The effectiveness of this work has been enhanced by the development of links with other interested bodies in which nurses play a role and which have an interest in nurses. Examples of this are EHMA and the European Public Sector Union (EPSU). This extends the range of information-gathering and the opportunity to collaborate with colleagues from other related disciplines to bring pressure to bear on European politicians.

While individuals are active on behalf of nursing in Europe, every nurse has a role to play in influencing policy formulation. Taking an active part is not as great a challenge as it may seem at first, and a first port of call should be the national representatives who form the constituency of such organizations. Some of these representatives are directly elected, for example, Members of the European Parliament (MEPs), while others determine international policy through local election (MPs). All are directly accessible through local surgeries and increasingly accessible via electronic media, especially email. The local lobbying of such representatives requires good information, and with the availability of documents through the Internet those wishing to take a more active role in the process can do so.

Another facet of this is the work that major organizations do to influence the different agendas in Europe. Major industries and businesses usually have or are part of lobbying groups. In the public sector, local authorities and universities usually have significant resources to monitor developments and generate responses. This is now reflected in various campaigns concerning healthy cities, healthy schools and employment regulations including pay and conditions. This gives Europe an immediacy which it often lacks when reported on the news. To influence policy through these various avenues it is important to appreciate that we are all Europeans now. The jibe that the UK constitutes the offshore islands is a response to the way in which the phrase 'European mainland' is used. Indeed, there is an argument that anything to do with the EU in particular should be handled as domestic rather than international policy.

To summarize, policy formulation in health care in general and nursing in particular can be haphazard. In recent years the profession has generated considerable resources, especially in those NNAs within the EU, to develop a proactive and not just a reactive response to policy formulation. The importance of active lobbying of local representatives who sit in these policy forums should not be underestimated, and nurses should ensure that they utilize the resources of their membership organizations. This will make sure that the widest range of views and opinions is available to influence agendas and their delivery.

Conclusion

There has been a long and successful history of nurses influencing policy formulation in Europe. It has survived as a process despite the vacillating nature of national politics. A real cohesion has developed among nurses, which is just as apparent when government chief nurses gather or expert practitioners in cancer care or occupational health meet. This unity of interest, which appears to be growing in the profession, is underlined by the increase in the number of European groups. These organizations are generating an increasing number of international events through which there is the real opportunity to learn about nursing in the wider context. It also reflects nurses' interest in sharing and growing together as a profession.

It is not easy to see why this should stop. The expansion of electronic communication media, and with it the availability of information, means that health care will be delivered in an environment where knowledge will be shared with service users, and health care professionals will increasingly facilitate choice rather than prescribe a single course of action. The impact of this on policy formulation will be significant indeed. It makes the notion of the global village a reality. If everyone has the opportunity to access available information simultaneously, then everyone will be able to vote simultaneously. This will be a return to the concept of democracy as practised in the city-states of ancient Greece, as all members of society will be able to contribute.

While many things might be decided by a majority vote, the need for knowledge generation will also increase. This will mean that policy formulation will operate in two directions at the same time. While organizational and national policies are being agreed, individuals will be in a position to change their practice or political position immediately. This immediacy will break down the last great barrier within Europe: concern about what is being done by the country next door. Without wishing to challenge notions of sovereignty, the availability of knowledge will reduce the likelihood that ignorance of colleagues in other countries will exercise its traditional bar to joint working and mutual understanding.

References

Commission of the European Communities (1988) *ACTN Report on Training in Cancer Nursing*, Brussels: CEC, Document III/D/248/3/88.

Commission of the European Communities (1994) *ACTN Report on the Guidelines for Education on Nursing Care of the Elderly*, Brussels: CEC, Document XV/E/8301/2/94.

Commission of the European Communities (2002) *Proposal for a Directive of the European Parliament and of the Council on the recognition of professional qualifications*, Brussels, COM (2002) 119 Final.

Council of Europe (1967) *The European Agreement on the Instruction and Education of Nurses*, Strasbourg: Council of Europe.

Council of Europe (1994) *European Health Committee, Working party on the role and education of nurses*, Strasbourg: Council of Europe.

Ludvigsen, C. and Roberts, K. (1996) *Health Care Policies and Europe – The implications for Practice*, Oxford: Butterworth-Heinemann.

Quinn, S. and Russell, S. (1993) *Nursing – The European Dimension*, London: Scutari.

Saltman, R.B. and Figueras, J. (1997) *European Health Care Reform – Analysis of Current Strategies*, WHO Regional Publications, European Series, No. 72, Copenhagen.

Treaty of Amsterdam amending the Treaty of European Union, the Treaties establishing the European Communities and certain related Acts, Luxembourg: The Office for Official Publications of the European Communities, 1998.

Treaty of European Union (The Maastricht Treaty), Luxembourg: The Office for Official Publications of the European Communities, 1992.

Woodham-Smith, C. (1950) *Florence Nightingale 1820–1910*, London: Constable.

World Health Organization (1989) *European Conference on Nursing*, Copenhagen: WHO Regional Office for Europe.

World Health Organization (1998) *Health For All for the Twenty-First Century – the Health Policy for Europe*, Geneva: WHO.
World Health Organization (2000) 'Nurses and midwives for health. A WHO European strategy for nursing and midwifery education', Copenhagen, WHO Regional Office for Europe (unpublished document EUR/00/5019309/15 for the Second WHO Ministerial Conference on Nursing and Midwifery in Europe, Munich, June).

5

Political Activity and the Nurse – A Professional Duty?

Marianne Arndt

Introduction

> The nurse shares with society the responsibility for initiating and supporting action to meet the health and social needs of the public. (ICN, 2000, p. 1)

These words of the International Council of Nurses' (ICN) ethical code appear under the heading 'Nurses and the people'. They leave no doubt that as professionals nurses have a duty that touches on political activities. However, the first ethical responsibility of nurses lies in excellent practice. Nursing as such has been identified as a moral action (Curtin, 1986; Johnson, 1994).

A number of mechanisms are in place in most countries to safeguard standards of practice and to ensure suitable education of students. These mechanisms are embedded in most health care systems and, in the main, nurses have considerable influence in their design and control. Nurses do not work in isolation, however, but invariably as members of a team within an institutional setting. It is appropriate, therefore, to examine the nurse's responsibility in relation to her influence on the prevailing institutional structures. Under the heading 'Nurses and the profession' the following statement is made in the ICN code:

> The nurse assumes the major role in determining and implementing acceptable standards of clinical nursing practice, management, research and education. The nurse is active in developing a core of research-based professional knowledge. The nurse, acting through the professional organisation, participates in creating and maintaining equitable social and economic working conditions in nursing. (ICN, 2000, p. 2)

Summary

This chapter deals with nurses' political responsibilities and action in general and with some of the aspects arising from the two ICN statements quoted above. First some general points about the relationship between politics and ethics will be made. This will be followed by an exploration of the role of various nursing organizations in the UK, Germany, Austria and Switzerland. In relation to the three German-speaking countries, first, the role of the professional organizations is examined in relation to their political involvement. Second, an educational perspective is presented, seen through the lens of political responsibility.

Politics and ethics

European countries have taken different routes to develop professional autonomy and self-regulation, and against the backdrop of diverse political and cultural givens, the politics of nursing presents a different picture in each country. Although in some countries, well-structured and formal arrangements are the norm, it may be that less rigid organizational environments allow greater leeway for unique and unconventional solutions to some of the impending problems of nursing which it seems are quite similar in most European countries. Questions such as the recognition of nurses, their professional status, education and involvement in decisions relating to health matters at local, national and international levels are shared across the UK and the European mainland. These questions are at once of a professional, ethical and political nature.

However, an ethical appreciation of nursing, which encompasses the above-mentioned political dimensions, is not simply undertaken by looking at the direct delivery of care or organizations representing nursing. Ethics in nursing should be viewed from a three-tiered perspective. I suggest looking at three areas of ethical responsibility and decision-making in order to understand the interrelationship of practice with politics (Arndt, 1996). Although these areas are interdependent, it is helpful to look at each one in turn.

The first area is the political one. Of course we are subject to the givens of our health care systems, and our external wellbeing depends much on the political situation in which we find ourselves. The financial state of a country influences health care expenditure. Similarly, war and natural catastrophes make a difference as to what can be offered in the way of health care. But within the overall political area there is little actual freedom in relation to individual action. Thus, in their role as citizens, nurses and patients share more or less the same duties and rights within this first area.

The second area can be identified as the institutional area. It will be apparent that both political and institutional aspects are dependent upon one another. Political decisions at the highest level will naturally influence the structure of any health care and social system as well as the diverse educational routes to becoming professionals in any such system.

Active engagement with professional issues appears to be a paramount responsibility of nurses with regard to this area. Within democratic institutional systems we have seen many changes over recent years, not only in the political arena, but also in the structures and practice of nursing. Documentation, care plans, standards of care and quality assurance are prominent concerns, and in-service education and career development have a high standing in nurses' consciousness.

Within the institutional area nurses have a responsibility to be interested in professional developments, to seek information and to take an active part in professional progress. In the UK, institutions such as the NMC (Nursing and Midwifery Council) and the RCN (Royal College of Nursing) guarantee that nurses themselves have power to direct the fate of nursing. Germany, Austria and Switzerland, on the other hand, have no statutory body in the sense of regulating education and career development. On the continent, in the three German-speaking countries these matters are the concern of the health authorities, which are governed by civil servants and medical doctors. Thus, even though structures may be well developed or just emerging, their impact on the delivery of care is indirect.

This brings us to the third area of ethical responsibility: the personal area. This aspect of the nurse's role is enacted where the everyday kind of decision-making takes place. It is indeed in this area where nurses are confronted directly with moral responsibility for everyday nursing actions. From this area moral authority grows. Even though external forces may limit the possibilities of action in many ways and institutional structures may assist or hinder, it is in the personal area that the therapeutic nursing relationship is lived. In this area personal values, high standards of professional conscientiousness, as well as personal and professional integrity, are called for. It can therefore be argued that the touchstone of excellent nursing practice is always at the point of direct delivery of care.

However, the not-free-to-be-moral debate has opened up further perspectives about this aspect of ethics in nursing. I refer to the seminal article by Swider, Yarling and McElmurray (1985) and to the scholarly debate this article has instigated (Yarling and McElmurray, 1986; Packard and Ferrara, 1988). The debate centres around the question how far a nurse's responsibility can be called upon in the face of a health care system, that negates the freedom of professional decision-making for nurses and does not proffer adequate resources for nursing.

Moral responsibility is shared throughout the three areas, and personal accountability may be said to be less as we move from the personal to the institutional and political areas. This does not mean that the individual nurse does not have to answer for structural mismanagement or political injustice. But it means that her personal accountability for the institutional environment in which she works is less than her moral accountability in the personal area. Also, it is further reduced as regards the political area, because as we move from the personal to the political, more people are involved in decision-making regarding policies, resource distribution, general structuring and overall financing. Nursing does not happen in a world of nursing, and therefore nurses are not solely responsible for the world in which they live. Nursing is part of a health care system that in turn is embedded within a system of social and civil services. These compete with each in any state for their position within the economy. However, nurses, as members of a profession, do share in public responsibility. This is the understanding which must precede any reading of the ICN code.

Nursing organizations

The UK

In the UK, a regulatory body responsible for nurse education, registration and professional conduct has been in operation since 1948. With the Nurses, Midwives, and Health Visitors Act of 1979 the British government delegated administrative powers to the United Kingdom

Central Council for Nurses, Midwives and Health Visitors (UKCC), and these powers have since been transferred to the new regulatory body, the Nursing and Midwifery Council (NMC) under another Act of Parliament, the Nursing and Midwifery Order 2001.

The new body is smaller than the UKCC and consists of 12 registrant members, 12 alternate registrant members and 11 lay members. The registrant members consist of equal numbers of nurses, midwives and health visitors. The lay members include people from education, employment and consumer groups.

The major function of the NMC is to establish and improve standards of nursing, midwifery and health visiting care in order to serve and protect the public. Its key tasks are to:

- maintain a register of all nurses, midwives and health visitors;
- develop standards and guidelines for nursing, midwifery and health visiting education, practice and conduct;
- provide advice for registrants on professional matters;
- ensure the quality of nursing and midwifery education;
- develop standards and guidance for the local supervision of midwives;
- consider both allegations of misconduct and unfitness to practise due to ill health.

For UK nurses, being struck off the professional register is a daunting possibility; it constitutes a major mechanism in ensuring safe practice, together with the Professional Conduct Committee, which considers allegations of misconduct. The NMC, like its predecessor the UKCC, issues various guidelines regarding professional conduct and advisory papers referring to specific areas of nursing practice (see also Pyne, 1991; Arndt, 1996).

In the UK, the 'professional organization' mentioned in the ICN code, is not the NMC, whose role is regulatory and statutory, but the Royal College of Nursing (RCN). The RCN is one of the largest professional nursing organizations in the world, and was founded in 1916. It boasts more than 340,000 members, which means that almost every second registered nurse is a member of this association. In addition there are other membership organizations, such as the Nurses' Christian Fellowship and the Catholic Guild of Nurses, which have much smaller memberships. Trade unions such as UNISON also have sections for nurses, and play a major role in promoting political awareness among nurses. Many members of the religiously or union-oriented organizations also hold RCN membership.

In a factsheet about the RCN, the following description is given:

> The RCN is independent and works with all political parties to improve standards of patient care. Working locally, nationally and internationally, the RCN promotes the interest of both individual nurses and of nursing as a profession through lobbying, media relations, conferences and publications. A registered charity, the RCN is a major contributor to the development of nursing practice and standards of care, as well as being a provider of higher and further education through the RCN Institute. (RCN, 1998)

Some of the political and professional activities undertaken by the RCN can be summarized as:

- promoting the interests of nurses and patients by working closely with the government, other unions and professional organizations, and voluntary bodies;
- offering guidance on pay and conditions;
- advising on legal matters;
- providing indemnity insurance for its members;
- providing education and professional development opportunities.

The RCN represents the UK at an international level and through it, UK nurses are affiliated to the ICN. Thus nurses in Britain are fortunate to have many aspects of their role and function firmly under the control of nurses.

Germany, Austria and Switzerland

In Germany, Austria and Switzerland the professional organizations play an important part as regards nursing and health care policies, legislation and education. In none of the three countries do professional bodies comparable to the NMC exist. All activities in which the professional organizations are engaged are stimulated by concerns emanating directly from nursing practice, and an individual's active involvement with a nursing organizations in all three countries is usually voluntary. Even for key activities, very few full-time positions exist. Nursing organizations more often than not have a president who does the political work in her spare time, in addition to working in a full- or part-time nursing post. This, however, is changing, and increasingly lead positions, with adequate secretarial support, are being created within many nursing organizations.

Germany

Hospital care

Traditionally, nursing in Germany is subject to a strong Christian influence. Health care institutions and hospitals have primarily been established and run by Catholic orders or by Protestant nursing congregations. To date about 50 per cent of all German health care institutions still belong to and are run by either Catholic or Protestant organizations. Forty per cent are financed and administered by regional or local governments. Most of these, however, were founded at the beginning of the nineteenth century as either Catholic or Protestant hospitals or as independent hospitals run by the Red Cross Association of Germany or by a variety of smaller welfare agencies. Other important suppliers of health care are the university teaching hospitals, which are also state-financed and about 10 per cent of the health care institutions are privately owned and run.

All institutions, be they private, Catholic or Protestant, are part of regional hospital requirement plans, administered and negotiated according to the principle of subsidiarity. Private, Catholic or Protestant hospitals as well as local state hospitals are run as independent, self-financing institutions although they receive negotiable government subsidies. Over and above this, all Catholic institutions are tied to the Catholic welfare organization Caritas and are thus connected to the Church.

Protestant institutions are either independent or linked to the national Protestant welfare foundation Diakonisches Werk. Other institutions are generally linked to either the Red Cross or the free welfare organization Paritätischer Wohlfahrtsverband. Most Protestant health care institutions are partly financed and administered by either a Protestant deaconess organization, of which there are several in different regions of Germany, or by individual parishes, while the Catholic institutions are run, financed and administered by Catholic nursing orders such as the Daughters of Charity (Sisters of St Vincent de Paul), the Brothers of Mercy or any of the numerous other orders which were founded in Europe during the eighteenth century. Individual parishes may also have their own hospital, nursing home, or community care centre. This last type of institution is often supplied through contract with nursing staff from one of the Catholic nursing orders.

The government hospital financing plan is constantly updated in collaboration with representatives from various provider organizations, the semi-private sick/health insurances, and the regional hospital associations (Krankenhausgesellschaft). The last combine voluntary expertise from within various fields of practice with professional economic expertise, using government funding but also creating income by consultative activities.

Community care

In Germany the situation in community care can only be understood in connection with the activities of the established nursing orders, the nursing congregations, the voluntary welfare agencies, and the Red Cross. Traditionally the church parishes, whether Catholic or Protestant, employed nurses to supply home care for the elderly and for the dying. Private nurses supplemented such services. In the mid-1970s community care services became the focus of the health care plans in the different regions. Local and regional governments offered financial support for community care and the same providers of hospital nursing began to establish community nursing centres. This caused considerable competition between Catholic, Protestant and Red Cross centres, which was intensified by the emergence of private nursing agencies. Such agencies established local, regional and national businesses, with many being run as small family businesses or cooperatives by enterprising nurses as well as by larger concerns, but with both employing nurses for the provision of home care.

In the old German Democratic Republic (GDR), all health care was controlled by the state, whether hospital or community based. Health centres were the focus of primary care and were augmented by clinical and community services. After the collapse of the GDR many nurses, especially those in the larger cities, ventured into establishing private nursing agencies. This development is continuing and presents one of the reasons for the renewed struggle for professional self-regulation. To date, with the approval of the local chambers of commerce, any person can set up a community nursing service but, in order to be successful, cooperation with general practitioners, local hospitals and the sickness insurance companies is a necessity. Generally contracts are developed between the insurers and any given provider as a basis for financial remuneration for care given.

Nursing education

Most hospitals have schools of nursing, and nursing education is regulated by federal law and complies with the European directives. Nurses in Germany undergo a three-year vocational course in one of the hospital schools. At present there is a movement to rationalize nurse education and to link smaller schools to form centralized institutions for nurse education. Some of these larger institutions are comparable to the former British colleges of nursing.

Nursing organizations in Germany

It is a complicated enterprise to describe the German nursing scene and to make it comprehensible to outside scrutiny. In order to enhance understanding of the political position of nursing, some historical peculiarities need to be highlighted. The deaconess movement initiated in Kaiserswerth near Düsseldorf by the Protestant pastor Theodor Fliedner and his wife Friederike promulgated the 'mother-house system' for nurses. Young, unmarried women were trained at Kaiserswerth before being sent to smaller institutions or into the community to carry out nursing work, as well as attend to the social and pastoral needs of patients. Generally the nurses stayed connected with the 'mother-house', which took care of them during periods of sickness and after their retirement. This system, which simultaneously provided both independence and security for women who did not marry, was adopted by new Protestant nursing congregations, founded throughout Europe (but mainly in Germany, Austria and Switzerland) and also by the Red Cross.

As the trained nurse became necessary for the advancement of medical science, administrators or medical directors of large university hospitals in Protestant areas invited these congregations or the Red Cross to draw up staffing contracts. Similarly, the need for nurses in Catholic areas was met by a variety of nursing orders.

The need for professional unity, and for financial independence of private nurses, led to the formation of a professional organization for nurses (Berufsorganisation der Krankenpflegerinnen, BO) by Agnes Karll in 1903. Agnes Karll (1868–1927) trained as a nurse within the security of the Red Cross mother-house system but became engaged in private nursing and quickly drew other nurses to her initially small organization.

The first world conference of the ICN in Berlin in 1904 took place at the invitation of the newly founded German professional organization. The ICN had been founded in London in 1899 during the Congress of the Women's World Federation. This provided the framework for the Annual Conference of the Matrons' Council of Great Britain, and Mrs Bedford-Fenwick was elected first president of the ICN. Agnes Karll was elected ICN president during the second world conference in London in 1909 (Mörgelin and Schwochert, 1997).

Karll's early endeavours to provide university education for nurses were thwarted by the First World War. However, she and her nursing colleagues were instrumental advisers of the Prussian government, which in 1908 passed the first nursing law in the German Reich. Here, for the first time, nursing matters were addressed from a legal perspective. Prerequisites for entry and training were legally stated. Other German states, such as Bavaria, Saxonia and Westphalia, modelled their developing nursing legislation on the Prussian law. It should be noted, however, that much legislation addressed the relationship between nursing and medicine especially at the time when new discoveries in the areas of microbiology and pharmacology meant that medicine's influence on everyday life was growing.

One important activity pursued by Agnes Karll was the provision for sickness insurance for self-employed nurses, as well as a pension scheme for retired nurses. Karll's organization was the forerunner of what is now the largest German nursing organization, the Deutscher Berufsverband für Krankenpflege (DBfK). The DBfK proved to be flexible and adaptable, and private hospitals with their own nurse training schools emerged. (Between 1954 and 1995 nurse teachers and nurse managers were educated to a very high standard at the Agnes Karll Institute for higher nurse education at Frankfurt.) The organization has about 20,000 members. It has always been respected in local and federal government quarters and was recognized as one of the partners with whom consultation regarding the structure of nursing and of nurse education was undertaken. (Renate Reimann, an internationally recognized nurse scholar, was the first director of an institution for further nurse education in Essen, Westphalia and initiated Germany's participation in nursing research with the WENR (Workgroup of European Nurse Researchers).) At present the DBfK is being reorganized, relinquishing some of its educational activities and forging a structure compatible with the new demands that have arisen from the unification of East and West Germany.

One of the foremost objectives is to provide for nurses' professional, political and personal empowerment by:

- contracted in-service education;
- organizing conferences;
- publishing one of the important German professional journals;
- representing nurses at regional and federal health care institutions.

Through the DBfK German nursing is linked to the International Council of Nursing (ICN).

Two Catholic associations are in existence, providing a spiritual and professional home for Catholic nurses who did not want to join a nursing order. In 1937 the nurse and social worker Adelheid Testa founded the Caritas nurses association (Caritas Gemeinschaft für Pflege- und Sozialberufe). It was linked to the Catholic Church via Caritas, the church's welfare organization. In 1959 the free Catholic professional association for nurses (Freier katholischer Berufsverband) was also formed as a competing organization.

Both organizations have established institutions for higher education in nursing where nurse teachers and nurse managers receive their education. Since 1992 these courses have been transferred to the Catholic universities for applied sciences (see note 10). All the Catholic nurses' associations are connected at an international level with CICIAMS (Comité International des Infirmières Catholiques et Assistantes Medico-Sociales) represented as a non-governmental organization (NGO) at the World Health Organization. Also connected with CICIAMS are various work groups of European Catholic nursing orders, which have members in Germany, Austria and Switzerland.

The mother-house system, established by the Protestant Church, although an important stepping-stone for women's emancipation, needed to be supplemented by independent nurses' organizations like their Catholic counterparts. Because of the Protestant denominational diversifications, numerous Christian nurses' associations were formed that did not require nurses to make a life commitment, unlike the deaconess movements. Of these associations the Protestant diacony association (Freier evangelischer Diakonieverband Zehlendorf) and the Kaiserswerth diacony association (Kaiserswerther Diakonieverband) are the largest surviving organizations. The Protestant organizations also run private institutions for higher nurse education, and many of these have recently transferred their activities to the tertiary level of education.

Other powerful groups in German nursing are the trade unions. The Trade Union for Public Services, Transport, and Traffic (ÖTV) has a nursing section and is very active in promoting political awareness among nurses. Also the German Employees' Association (DAG) hosts a nursing section. Both trade unions together run about twenty centres for further nurse education. As such, they provided most of Germany's post-qualification education before the advent of academic courses for nurse teachers and nurse managers. In comparison, the Red Cross has one institute, while the Catholic and Protestant organizations together have seven institutes offering post-qualification courses. These latter institutions, however, have transferred some longer courses into the tertiary education sector.

A further trade union activity specific to nursing should be mentioned. In 1991, 115 German nurses from the South Western regions founded their own nursing trade union, Gewerkschaft Pflege (GP), which is open to nurses from all branches of nursing. Its aim is to foster public interest in nursing issues by highlighting problems related to working conditions and salaries (Benn-Roloff, 1997). It offers consultation services for nurses, workshops on ethical and legal issues, and organizes congresses. Membership has increased all over Germany and currently is in excess of 1,800.[1]

The confusing diversity of German political activities in the area of nursing has a healthy competitive element. All organizations are consulted at local, regional and federal levels by government commissions, and their representatives attend hearings and have opportunities to promote nursing from their specific perspectives. All organizations publish their own professional journals.

Three further organizations in particular have a powerful influence on structuring nursing's future in Germany. These are the work group representing nurse managers, Bundesarbeitsgemeinschaft leitender Krankenpflegepersonen (BALK); the commission of nurse teachers Bundesausschuß der Lehrer- und Lehrerinnen für Krankenpflege (BALLK); and the organization for private nursing services in the community, Arbeitgeberverband ambulanter Pflegedienste (AVAP).

Unity in diversity

The overall membership in German professional nursing organizations is small when compared with RCN membership in the UK. A rough calculation of members across the various organizations amounts to about 10 per cent of the nursing population. It is often nurses in leading or teaching positions who are active members of such organizations. Thus there is an active nucleus of professionals concerned and involved in the democratic structures of political decision-making.

Discussion and consultations about issues affecting nursing at federal political levels are invariably prepared by local and regional hearings, where representatives from all organized groups are invited by the respective government ministerial officers to forward opinions, statements or programmed solutions to the problems at hand. This forces the members of the various organizations into an ongoing debate and produces a high level of political awareness. Increasingly of late, joint conferences have been held and joint councils formed, enabling joint statements to be issued.

Such collaborative activities are not new but have a long history in German nursing. In 1953 the first decisive effort was made to improve communication between the different factions in the German nursing world. The work group of German nursing associations, Arbeitsgemeinschaft Deutscher Schwesternschaften und Pflegeorganisationen (ADS) was founded, of which the German Red Cross nursing association is an important member. A Catholic, Protestant, or a Red Cross nurse representative takes the chair of this work group on a rotational basis and various joint publications of political importance have been released over the years. For instance, a paper on the rights and duties of nurses regarding venepuncture was produced, and more importantly statements on nurse education have strongly influenced state legislation.

Regular meetings and debates between the steering committee of the DBfK, the largest free nursing association, and the ADS have now found an organizational structure. In June 1998 a German Nursing Council, Deutscher Pflegerat (DPR), was established. Other organizations include the German Midwives' Federation, the German Professional Association of Geriatric Nurses, the German Professional Association of Paediatric Nurses, and the German Federation of Male Nurses. These groups are all members of the new council, DPR.

This has meant concerted action on a number of fronts, such as the identification of professional and political issues and problems in nursing, analysis of facts and figures, international comparisons of nursing situations, and suggestions for future developments in nursing.

Unification

Following unification in 1990 it was apparent that Catholic as well as Protestant organizations had survived the Communist regime. The Caritas Nurses' Association had continued to exist within the German Caritas Association, and contacts between East and West German groups were kept alive by frequent visits. After retirement, East German nurses regularly visited Freiburg, where the headquarters of the Caritas Nurses' Association is located, and undercover training was provided to East German Catholic nurses between the 1950s and the 1980s under the guise of visiting relatives. Caritas nurses held seminars in private homes to update nurses on professional topics and thus kept personal as well as professional contacts alive. One of the greatest difficulties for this work was the fact that no printed material, such as lecture notes, was allowed to cross the border from West to East. This meant that no books, no teaching aids and no scripts could be taken to these seminars. Teaching content had to be memorized and teaching generally took the form of discussion and debate.

Even though no official contact was permitted between organizations, individual members of the Red Cross, the Protestant groupings, the DBfK, and the trade unions kept in contact with East German colleagues throughout the time of the GDR. After unification the different groupings extended their activities into eastern regions and thus contributed to the restructuring of the 'Neue Länder' (the provinces of the former GDR).

Politics and nurse education in Germany

In 1986 the directors of the German institutions for further education formed a standing committee[2] concerned with political, structural and curricular issues in nursing and nurse education. Connections with comparable institutions in Austria and in Switzerland were made which proved to be of great importance to international exchange between the German-speaking countries. Nursing leaders in key positions and from various backgrounds met for these discussions. Until this time, it had not been easy for nurses from Catholic, Protestant, trade union, Red Cross or independent nursing associations to meet, as traditionally members of these institutions were at variance and open debate was avoided. However, growing political awareness in Germany, in the wake of the 1977 European directives regarding nursing and nursing legislation, demanded greater cohesion by the different nursing representatives if nursing was to speak with one voice.

Two years later the German Association for the Furtherance of Nursing Science and Nursing Research (DV)[3] was founded as an outgrowth of the standing committee. This committee has since dissolved, and the deans of nursing departments in the various universities and universities for applied sciences, together with their nursing representatives, have formed a 'Deans' Conference', which is pursuing similar objectives. These are: to establish nursing education firmly in German academia; to ensure the comparability of structures and content in the different academic establishments; and to raise points for debate. The Deans' Conference meets two or three times a year and has bolstered serious discussions on the academic future of nursing in Germany. The ideological differences, which in former times prevented contact between various factions, no longer act as a barrier to progress. Political issues involved in the establishment and furthering of nursing as a discipline have become key aspects of the debate, while the differences between the various groups may serve as competitive incentives to push for academic accreditation.

The DV meanwhile has about 500 members and has developed many activities in all fields of nursing and nursing science, including ethics. This association is independent, and one of its great achievements has been to bring together the diversified interests in German nursing on the basis of developing nursing as a discipline. It also has active theme groups and sections whose members pursue their interests in a variety of areas, such as history, teaching nursing science at the tertiary level, and ethics. Many of its members are nurse teachers, lecturers at one of the universities, or students in post-qualification programmes. Members meet three or four times a year and they publicize and hold symposia.

Traditionally nurse teachers in Germany attend an eighteen-month to two-year full-time course at one of the larger institutions, as do nurse managers. Recently teacher and manager preparation has been moved into academia. This process started tentatively in 1980 with the Katholische Fachhochschule in Osnabrück,[4] incorporating a nurse teacher as well as a nurse manager programme into its Faculty of Social Sciences. Until 1997 no degree was awarded, but a certificate was issued to students successfully completing the course. Meanwhile about forty Universities for Applied Sciences offer teaching and management degree courses for nurses. The State Fachhochschule in Osnabrück was the first to offer a management degree in nursing in 1986; and was first to establish a chair of nursing and social science, occupied by Ruth Schröck as the first professor of nursing in Germany. The various courses are full- or part-time and are comparable to an honours degree. They are approved by respective Ministry of Education in each of the Länder.

So far only four traditional universities offer nursing degree programmes. Three of these (Humboldt University of Berlin, Free University of Bremen and University of Halle) also offer a degree course for nurses teachers and the University of Hamburg offers a degree course for teachers in health care sciences, which attracts nurses and midwives, as well as dietitians, physiotherapists and occupational therapists. The private University of Witten-Herdecke offers the only degree in nursing science in Germany as a pilot programme organized initially over six semesters (three years) resulting in a bachelor's degree. Following a further four semesters of study, a candidate can gain a master's degree in nursing.

German legislation relating to tertiary education stipulates direct entry to academic institutions if educational requirements are fulfilled. This means that it is possible for school-leavers who fulfil university entry requirements to have access to nurse teacher degrees or management courses without needing to have gained a basic nursing qualification. Although possible, it is difficult for institutions to bypass these regulations and therefore some universities require at least a minimum of six months' practical nursing experience.

German unification gave a huge boost to the movement of nursing into academia. Humboldt University in Berlin and the University of Halle, both in the former German Democratic Republic (GDR), had a long history of offering university courses for teachers in the health care professions. Despite a great many institutions of the former GDR being dismantled after unification in 1990, these universities managed to retain the health care teacher courses. With some substantial changes in personnel and content, nursing science was introduced and these universities now boast the longest academic tradition in nursing.

Immediately after unification many West German nurses enrolled with the Humboldt and Halle Universities, taking advantage of their first opportunity to gain a nursing-related degree. Restructuring in the former GDR also resulted in the foundation of a number of new universities for applied sciences, and most of these immediately included nurse teacher and management degree courses in their programmes. So far, however, no generic pre-registration nursing programmes have been offered, so that basic nurse education is still tied to hospital schools.

Austria

Austrian Nurses' Association

In Austria there is no equivalent to the UK statutory body, the NMC, and no registration system exists. Legislation in relation to nursing is found within general health legislation, employment legislation and specific nursing law. The local medical authorities are responsible for ensuring a high standard of nurse education and they supervise qualification procedures.

The situation in Austria regarding professional organizations presents a more unified picture than that in Germany. The first Austrian nursing association was founded 1884 by the Viennese surgeon, Billroth. Following this, in 1933 Austrian nurses formed a nursing union, which became a member of the ICN (Editorial, 1988). This was the predecessor of the Austrian Nurses' Association Österreichischer Krankenpflegeverband (ÖKV), which today has over 10,000 members, representing some 25 per cent of Austrian nurses.

Each of the nine Austrian regions boasts a regional sector of the association with its own president, who is generally a part-time employee of the ÖKV working as a nurse, nurse teacher or nurse manager. The national president leads the organization and is aided by a full-time nurse and a secretary. It is important to note that it is only since 1997 that the president of the ÖKV has held a full-time position. Until then the presidency was an honorary position. ÖKV operates on the basis of political independence and interconfessional membership.[5] The 'political' objectives of the Austrian association are ethically grounded. The following statement forms the basis for all activities of the ÖKV:

The ÖKV holds that the basis for all nursing activities is the respect for life and human dignity as well as recognition of the basic human rights. Therefore the ÖKV aims to assure that, independent of ideology, political conviction, nationality, race, age, sex and social position, everyone in need of nursing care and nursing assistance has a right to such care and assistance.[6]

The objectives of the ÖKV include:

- development of nurse education at pre-registration and post-qualification levels;
- enhancement of personality development of its members and preservation and furtherance of the good reputation of the nursing profession;
- furthering the advancement of nursing by publications of professional interest (publication of a professional journal as well as statements related to nursing practice);
- representation of nurses' professional and social interests;
- involvement with health promotion and health education in all areas of the health care services;
- improving the working conditions of nurses in Austria.

Political activities of the Austrian Nurses' Association

An important aspect of the ÖKV's political involvement is the continuous struggle for independence of the nursing profession. In 1994 the Austrian government held an official inquiry as to the independence, accountability and responsibility of the nursing profession. The political involvement of nurses was documented by active participation of nursing representatives from the ÖKV, the Austrian Association of Health Care Workers, representatives of the Austrian Workgroup of Nursing Directors, as well as the Association of Religious Nursing Orders in Austria; members of the inquiry commission also included medical doctors, and this debate is ongoing.

The ÖKV has also been instrumental in developing the new federal nursing law, which was adopted in 1997. Here, the role of the qualified nurse has been defined as:

- independent regarding nursing actions;
- jointly responsible for medical/nursing activities;
- interdisciplinary-oriented.

Representatives of the organization are involved in consultative procedures regarding all legislation relevant to health care. Furthermore, representatives sit on government expert health care planning committees as well as being involved with the Austrian Federal Institute for Health Issues.

Nurse representatives of the ÖKV are also involved in the development of nursing curricula at the highest federal and at regional levels of governement.

Members of the ÖKV can use an advisory service for legal and professional matters, and members experiencing problems with the implementation of nursing legislation in practice situations receive professional and legal advice in relation to their personal situation. One example of the importance of involvement in legal aspects is the expert verdict given by the ÖKV in January 1999.[7] This involved a nursing director who had reorganized night duties in a residential nursing home. About fifty-five of the 100 patients in the home needed specialized care such as dialysis or percutaneous entero-gastrostomy (PEG) feeding. Some patients also needed qualified supervision. Previously two care assistants had covered the night duty rota. This was changed so that one qualified nurse and one care assistant would in future be employed. The case caused substantial internal upset in the home about the level of qualifications needed to provide nursing care in specific circumstances. An expert verdict was procured by the ÖKV and this is now being used all over Austria to demonstrate the legal, professional and personal accountability and responsibility of qualified nurses, nursing directors and care assistants. In the verdict it was made evident that all three groups can and must act solely on the basis of their qualification, and for special nursing care a qualified nurse needs to be employed. Further, nursing directors must ensure such employment and all nursing care delivered must be transparent by the use of:

- nursing assessment (compiling information about a patient which will be used to establish a care plan, establishing the degree of dependence of a patient on nursing interventions);
- nursing diagnosis (being the basis for professional judgement as to nursing problems and as to the cause of such problems, as well as a further basis for care planning);
- nursing care plan (including nursing outcomes and nursing interventions);

- nursing action (including appropriate documentation);
- evaluation of nursing actions (used for assessment of the effectivity of care and for reassessment of nursing needs).

Further, the verdict clearly stated that the qualified nurse holds independent responsibility for

- the documentation of care planning;
- giving (to patients and relatives) information on disease prevention and health education;
- adequate psychosocial care;
- organization of care delivery services;
- supervision and instruction of assisting personnel;
- supervision and teaching of nursing students.

This verdict provides a legal and a moral background for nursing practice and is of substantial political importance. Here a nurse used her professional judgement in the organization of services and, not being satisfied, sought the political backing of her professional organization. The expert verdict ensures the legal standing of qualified nurses and of nurse supervisors. This situation is also important as it demonstrates the possibility for cooperation between a professional organization and the legal profession without the need for elaborate structures. The important factors in this situation included the personal and professional courage which enabled the director to stand up for the needs of patients; and the support given by the national organization in procuring an expert verdict.

Nursing and higher education in Austria

Several Austrian institutions offer further education and degree courses for nurses. At the University of Graz an ordinary degree course in public health is available for nurses may follow, and the degree programme for educational sciences offers some seminars relevant to nursing. The Institute for Higher Nurse Education (Mödling) in conjunction with the University of Vienna offers an associate university certificate for nurse teachers and for nursing management.

At the Institute for Higher Nurse Education in Mödling qualified nurses with three years' practical experience in any field of nursing can follow a two-year full-time university course to qualify as nurse teachers or managers, and similar courses have been introduced at Salzburg, Linz and Innsbruck.

In most parts of Austria nurse training takes place in the traditional hospital schools, run either locally or regionally by the state, or by various Catholic nursing and teaching orders. They are generally attached to a hospital or a hospital group. An exception is found in the German-speaking Bozen (Bolzano) or Tyrol, which is administratively part of Italy. Italian legislation requires schools of nursing to be independent institutions of higher education. Tyrolean nurses and nurse teachers had generally been part of the Austrian nursing scene but from 1997, the Bolzano school of nursing became part of the Fachhochschule, the university for applied sciences in Bolzano, so that Tyrolean nurses' basic education is conducted at an academic level.

As nursing is not an academic subject in Austria, many nurses, nurse teachers and managers take master's degrees in related subjects such as educational sciences, psychology, sociology, philosophy, politics and history, or business studies and economics. Thus, in Austria nursing leaders are increasingly well prepared to join the political debates related to the future structures of nursing, nursing education and nursing's role within the health services.

Switzerland

Swiss nursing organizations

In Switzerland, as in other European countries, the origins of organized nursing go back to the women's movements of the late 1800s. The Swiss Charitable Women's Organization had a nursing commission in 1896 and the first organized structure emerged in the Kanton of Zürich in 1909, when 40 private nurses joined forces to increase employment security. In 1910 the predecessor of today's Swiss Nursing Association, Schweizer Berufsverband für Krankenschwestern und Krankenpfleger (SBK), was founded.

The objectives of this federation were the furtherance of public recognition of nursing by the provision of guidelines for nurses' uniforms, nurses' salaries and conditions of service, as well as providing further education for experienced nurses. A further objective was met with the institution of a sickness and welfare insurance scheme and an old age pension for retired nurses.

In order to ensure national unity in the education of health care professionals, the cantons entrusted the supervision of basic nurse education to the Swiss Red Cross in 1909, and throughout the years, befitting Swiss culture, the organization issued both German and French nursing publications with the aim of informing and educating.

Evidence of an early interest in professional politics as well as in research was provided by initiating a study of the activities of nurses and the nursing needs of patients. Begun in 1965, the study was conducted by a nurse with the help of an expert from WHO. It was jointly supported by the Swiss Red Cross, the cantons, the Swiss Hospitals' Association and the Swiss Nurses' Association.

Swiss nurses were heavily involved with the international work of the ICN, which Switzerland joined in 1937. In 1966 the headquarters of the ICN moved to Geneva, and the then executive director was a member of the Swiss Nurses' Association.

In 1978 a joint association was formed, the Schweizer Berufsverband der Krankenschwestern und Krankenpfleger, SBK.[8] One of the special features of nursing in Switzerland has been the separate basic training for psychiatric and paediatric nurses. This resulted in these groups founding their own associations. The structure was changed with the reform of basic education in 1991.

The Swiss Nurses' Association today

The SBK to date[9] has over 25,000 members. This represents approximately 30 per cent of the Swiss nursing population. Because the Swiss federal system allows each canton to have its own health laws and services, the SBK has thirteen chapters. This allows it to engage in local and cantonal health policy-making as well as developmental and union activities. Thus some of the chapters use French, German, Italian or Rhaeto-Romanic as their main language, and the monthly nursing journal displays linguistic parity.

The main aim of the SBK is to develop nursing and the quality of care, to strengthen and further the nursing profession, to improve working conditions for nurses and to promote and support the membership in professional activities and development. From its very beginning one of the main objectives has been a commitment to further education. The SBK regulates and supervises specialist courses in intensive care, theatre nursing, anaesthetic nursing and clinical specialisms. Also, the Association is involved with basic education at decision-making levels.

The organizational structure of the SBK supports full-time posts as well as nurses from all areas of nursing practice who hold honorary and advisory positions. The headquarters of the organization, with three main divisions (education, nursing and professional politics), is in Bern. Connected with the SBK is an Institute for Nursing Research in Bern and two centres for further education, in Zürich and Lausanne. Several expert commissions are involved in questions related to research, ethics and education. Work groups concern themselves with specific issues related to the various fields of nursing and nurse education.

The following services are offered to members:[10]

• advice on all employment queries;
• legal protection;
• financial assistance in professional and social emergency situations;
• bursaries and loans for courses of study at home and abroad;
• involvement with research projects;
• reduction of congress and course fees;
• a monthly nursing journal.

Membership also guarantees democratic participation in developing the future of nursing as well as sickness insurance, credit cards, reduced-price language courses, and reduced-price pharmaceutical products.

The SBK is politically active in many areas and has consultative status in legislative procedures related to health issues. Members are informed about current issues that may impinge on the professional identity of nurses, on political questions that have implications for health care, and, before public opinion polls, which are held frequently by the Swiss government, the SBK publishes position papers. For example, a dossier was prepared by the SBK on the following question to all Swiss citizens:

> Should Switzerland sign the European Convention on Human Rights in Biomedicine?

Nursing at tertiary level in Switzerland

Traditionally Swiss nurse teachers as well as nurse managers qualified at two schools for higher education run by the Swiss Red Cross, one in Lausanne for French-speaking nurses and one in Aarau for German-speaking nurses (Weiterbildungszentrum für Gesundheitsberufe WE'G–SRK). Teacher training courses will be offered at degree level; the qualification aimed at will be equivalent to that offered by a Fachhochschule.

In February 2000, the Institute of Nursing Science, with a professorial chair in Nursing Science, opened at the University of Basel and a Master's in Nursing Science commenced in October 2000. This is an important political step for the development of nursing as an academic discipline in the German-speaking countries of Europe.

Meanwhile – August 2003 – a number of changes regarding the educational system for health care professionals have taken place. Legislation has been passed as to the integration of nursing education at the tertiary diploma level. General prerequisite for this type of three-year course is the 'Matura' certificate (equivalent to A-levels in all relevant subjects). The course is a modular one and is comparable to other courses in the Swiss educational system at the same level leading to professional qualifications. The official title of those having passed the course and being enabled to independently function as first level nurses will be 'DiplomPflege-Fachfrau/Fachmann' (Diploma as a Specialist in Nursing).

An important feature of the new system is the possibility to grant access to the course through a variety of routes. Apart from the full *Matura* it will be possible to access by specialized exams in the social and health-care sciences at A-level grades (Berufsmatura). Further, a newly created occupation is the 'Fachangestellte-Gesundheit (FAGE)' Qualified Health-Care-Employee). After having obtained a basic school-leaving certificate a student may enter a three-year course leading to the FAGE qualification. This entails the possibility to work as nursing assistant under the supervision of a fully qualified nurse and it allows access to the nurse education proper. It also opens access to other professional health care courses leading to qualifications such as Occupational Therapist, Physiotherapist, or Radiology Assistant.

The Swiss Red Cross is no longer responsible for structure and implementation of educational development in the health care professions. Meanwhile the 'Bundesamt für Berufsbildung und Technologie' (Federal Office for Professional Education and Technology) has taken over here.

Information: www.sbk-asi.ch

Conclusion

In this chapter an overview has been given of some of the important issues in nursing in the three German-speaking countries. The role of the various nursing organizations has been shown to be key in ensuring that the political involvement of nurses is part and parcel of everyday nursing life.

Notes

1. Personal communication from the founding president of the GP.
2. Ständige Konferenz der Leiterinnen und Leiter der Fort- und Weiterbildungsinstitute für Krankenpflege im deutschsprachigen Raum.

3. Deutscher Verein für die Förderung von Pflegewissenschaft und -forschung (DV).
4. 'Fachhochschule' (FHS) will be translated hereafter by University for Applied Sciences'. This term is already being used officially in the title of a number of such academic institutions. A Fachhochschule is classed as an academic establishment but without the right to award doctoral degrees. In a way FHS are comparable to the new universities in Britain, formerly polytechnic colleges.
5. Personal communication from the current president of the ÖKV.
6. Author's translation from ÖKV information material.
7. Allmer/January 1999 Die Eigenverantwortlichkeit in der Gesundheits- und Krankenpflege unter besonderer Berücksichtigung der Pflegehilfe. This verdict is available from the Österreichischer Krankenpflegeverband, 1182 Vienna, Postfach 63, Mollgasse 3a, Austria.
8. This information stems from written communications from the SBK secretarial section, Professional Politics (Bern, 7 May 1999).
9. Figures are taken from the SBK annual report 1997, p. 27.
10. From an information brochure of the SBK.

References

Arndt, M. (1996) *Ethik denken – Maßstäbe zum Handeln in der Pflege*, Stuttgart: Georg Thieme Verlag.

Benn-Roloff, N. (1997) 'Strikes – an appropriate action for health care employees? A personal perspective', *Nursing Ethics*, **4** (4): 339–342.

Curtin, L.L. (1986) 'The Nurse as Advocate: A Philosophical Foundation for Nursing', in Chinn, P.L. (ed.) *Ethical Issues in Nursing*, Rockville, MD: Aspen Systems, pp. 11–20.

Editorial (1988) '40 Jahre österreichischer Krankenpflegeverband', *Österreichische Krankenpflegezeitschrift*, **6** (7): 164–167.

International Council of Nurses (2000) *The ICN Code of Ethics for Nurses*, Geneva: ICN.

Johnson, J. (1994) 'A dialectical examination of nursing art', *Advances in Nursing Science*, **17**: 1–14.

Mörgelin, K. and Schwochert, B. (1997) *Pflege in Europa von A bis Z*, Eschborn: DBfK Bundesverband.

Packard, J.S. and Ferrara, M. (1988) 'In search of the moral foundations of nursing', *Advances in Nursing Science*, **10**: 60–71.

Pyne, R.H. (1991) *Professional discipline in nursing*, 2nd edn, London: Blackwell Scientific Publications.

Royal College of Nursing (1998) 'Factsheet: About the Royal College of Nursing', London: RCN.

Swider, S.A., Yarling, R.R. and McElmurry, B.J. (1995) 'Ethical decision making in a bureaucratic context by senior nursing students', *Nursing Research*, **34**: 108–112.

Yarling, R.R. and McElmurry, B.J. (1986) 'The moral foundation of nursing', *Advances in Nursing Science*, **8**: 63–75.

6

Interprofessional Relationships: Collaboration or Confrontation?

Maria Gasull

Introduction

Social, economic and technical changes that have occurred in recent decades have had a profound effect on society in general and on health care in particular. Technological advances have enabled many illnesses that were previously fatal to be cured. The consequences have been many and, in general, the results positive, as can be seen in longer life expectancies and improved wellbeing of many western populations. These factors, together with changing public expectations, have caused politicians, economists and especially health professionals to examine their roles and introduce new systems of working that are better suited to the changing circumstances. The process of adaptation to these new realities has resulted in new professions being created and has meant that those in existence have had to rethink and reconstruct their functions and methods of working.

Summary

The chapter begins by exploring the concept of teamwork and the evolution of professions. It considers the characteristics of a profession, highlighting the popular debate as to whether nursing has successfully been transformed from a skilled occupation to a profession.

The chapter goes on to examine the doctor–nurse relationship, drawing on the work of Stein (1967) and considers why earlier nurses may have perpetuated the game before exploring why nurses now refuse to play, and the effect this has had on doctor–nurse relationships.

This is followed by an account of the various research studies on doctor–nurse relationships before examining the prerequisites for successful interprofessional relationships. The state of such relationships is then explored in the contexts of Spain and the United Kingdom. Finally it is argued that successful interprofessional relationships require more than dialogue and collaboration. In particular, they depend upon moral attitudes of trust, mutual respect and responsibility.

Teamwork

The explosion of knowledge that came about during the last century has made it impossible for a single professional to possess all the knowledge and abilities necessary to cure or treat an individual with a particular illness. Rather, it is necessary for different professionals, with a range of knowledge and expertise, to work together to achieve the same objectives, in what nowadays is known as the multidisciplinary team approach.

Today, no one doubts the importance of teamwork, but, in spite of the apparent universal acceptance of its importance in current health care, it is also true that many problems arise as a result of human relations.

To work as part of a team is not easy. It means being in contact with other human beings, working with people who may not always share the same values or ideals, and who, of course, will have different personalities. Although such people are trained to work together, positive outcomes are not guaranteed. It can be difficult, for example, to determine who exercises authority within the team, how such authority will be implemented, and how the different areas of responsibility of the professionals are to be defined.

Within the world of health care, teamwork is essential. In order to be able to cover health needs and make sure that patients are treated in the best possible manner, qualified health professionals such as doctors, nurses, physiotherapists and so on are required to work in a way which provides cover for 24 hours per day, 365 days per year. This, of course, makes working as a team especially difficult.

Doctors and nurses have formed the basic health care team, working together to maintain the population's good health and cure those who are ill. Their relationships with one another have undergone various changes due to the way in which their respective professions have evolved. It is interesting to make a historical analysis (Gracia, 1998, p. 12), since health and illness are not merely natural facts of life but are historical phenomena, as are the resultant related areas of knowledge, professional development and professional practices. The world of health care is an enormous, human creation which can only be fully understood within a historical context.

The evolution of professions

For centuries only the judge, doctor and priest were considered true professionals, while other workers belonged to the group know as 'skilled workers'. The professionals were admired, as life and law depended on them. They were powerful and enjoyed impunity, as well as many privileges. They were deemed by society to be 'excellent', a privilege that other skilled workers did not enjoy. They possessed high moral esteem and were in danger of misusing their paternalistic tendencies, obliging others to obey them as a son would obey a father.

Most changes in the concept of profession took place during the twentieth century. Judges, doctors and priests have gradually become more democratic, losing both some of their privileges and impunity. Increasingly they have had to comply with the same laws as other citizens and skilled workers. The law applies equally to each individual and, little by little, many differences between the ways in which the traditional professionals and other members of society were treated have disappeared. The role and function of each occupation have become more clearly defined, and their legal and moral responsibilities more established. It could be said that the concept of profession is not limited to the three aforementioned roles, but that the vast majority of occupations are also considered as professions. Problems only arise when the professional space or area of practice has to be defined, as this is linked to the allocation of power, which can cause continual conflict (Gracia, 1998).

Characteristics of professional activity

Various authors have studied the prerequisites for a human activity to be considered a profession (Jolley and Allan, 1992). Arroyo *et al.* (1997) outlines a model involving a large range of characteristics to enable us to understand exactly what constitutes a profession, what its moral features are, and how the account can be applied to the nursing profession. They define a profession as those occupational activities that include the following features:

1. A profession is an activity that provides society with a specific service in a institutionalized manner. This service must comprise the following characteristics:

    (a) the service must be unique, whereby professionals claim the right to lend their services exclusively.
    (b) the service to be provided must be clearly defined. The public must be informed of what they may expect to receive and what they may demand.
    (c) this must be treated as an indispensable task, a service which society cannot do without, without losing the right to health.

2. The profession is considered as kind of vocation and mission; for this reason the professional who dedicates himself to his profession is expected to invest time in preparation for this task.
3. Professionals exercise their profession in a stable manner, obtaining from it their means of earning a living and considering each other as colleagues.
4. Professionals form part a collective body who try to gain monopolistic control in carrying out their profession.
5. The profession may be exercised only after a thorough theoretical and practical training, that is by following a clearly set out course of studies, whereby a license or credentials are awarded on successful completion. The profession of nursing is now recognized as satisfying these criteria and is therefore considered as belonging to this body.
6. Professionals require an autonomous atmosphere in which to exercise their profession. They are the experts at what they do and it is they who are best suited to deciding what is professionally correct. It is necessary to establish a balance between the rights of the population to receive quality care without being over demanding, and the judgements of the experts who possess the knowledge

and means without becoming corporate. That is why associations and professional colleges establish professional codes for auto-regulation and in order to resolve conflicts.

7. The word *autonomy* also implies assuming the *responsibility* that is inherent to exercising the profession [see Scott's chapter following]. (Arroyo *et al.*, 1997, 22–24)

On analysing the aforementioned characteristics it can be seen that nursing has begun the transformation from a skilled job to a profession, and that the question as to whether it should or should not be deemed a profession no longer arises. What is not so clear, however, is whether this transformation has been fully realized. There are various criteria and opinions as to how such a conversion should be undertaken and which processes should be adopted (Jolley and Allan, 1992).

On reviewing the literature on nursing and the process of professionalization, it is apparent that this is a topic to which the nursing profession has dedicated much attention and one over which considerable controversy continues to be generated on both sides of the Atlantic. Sceptics might suggest that only those who are insecure look to status and make frequent use of the term 'to be members of a profession'. One possible reason for such a sizeable literature on this subject is that nursing has not yet acquired full professional status, although it has traditionally been given this title and some current writers prefer to classify nursing as an emerging profession, or semi-profession.

Doctor–nurse relationship

Of all the professional relationships within health care, perhaps the most important and permanent is that between nurses and doctors. People, both healthy and ill, consider them as essential members of the health care team and demand that they work as a team. Curtin (1982) explains how the nurse is an ever-present element and how, through her, patients and their relatives are able to have direct contact with the health system. The nurse is also the person with whom patients and relatives communicate more freely and sincerely. In spite of this, however, nurses may be considered by patients and relatives, as well as by other health professionals, including doctors, as inferiors rather than as colleagues. The reasons for these conceptions can probably be found in the history of the medical and nursing professions.

Early literature on nursing ethics or the professional duties of the nurse frequently describes her role as one of obedience and submission. Even quite recently in historical terms Stein (1967) wrote a seminal paper on the doctor–nurse relationship. He describes the relationship as a game, 'the doctor–nurse game'. This game, he claims, is an intricate model of conduct where one is able to perceive medical dominance and an attitude of deference and respect on the part of the nurse. Any interaction is carefully executed to prevent disturbing the hierarchical equilibrium. Nurses may be brave, they may take the initiative and make recommendations concerning patient care, but they must always appear to be passive. To put this another way, nurses can have ideas, make suggestions – even decisions – which are expected of them, but to all intents and purposes it must appear as though the doctor is responsible for any initiative. For many years nurses have kept up this game for a variety of reasons. Curtin and Flaherty (1982) and Fagin (1992) have suggested reasons for this phenomenon as follows:

1. The training received by the nurse was inferior to that of doctors so that their knowledge and qualifications did not permit them to work under the same conditions.
2. Historically, society demanded that women were submissive and obedient and that men were responsible for making decisions.
3. Nurses' working conditions were inferior and administrative policies made obedience easier.

This game has undergone some changes during recent years and in 1990, Stein and his collaborators reviewed their account of the doctor–nurse relationship (Stein *et al.*, 1990). They observed that great changes had taken place in the working relationship. On the one hand, it appeared that doctors were no longer held in such high esteem by the public, and that their 'omnipotence', which had always been present, was now disappearing as society no longer considered them infallible. On the other hand, they recognized that nurses had unilaterally decided not to play 'the doctor–nurse game' any longer. This was due to a number of reasons, including: a growing awareness of their progress towards recognition and achievement of professional autonomy, and a willingness to assume responsibilities and obligations arising from their growing autonomy. Also, both the feminist and human rights movements have played a part in increasing gender equality, making it easier for women to reject the passive, submissive and obedient role imposed by society. Nurses have acquired confidence, which has enabled them to improve their working conditions. At the same time, doctors have lost some of their public recognition and professional power, resulting in changing working relationships. Stein also indicated that doctors, in general, have ignored changes with respect to nurses, so that their general lack of awareness of change left them feeling betrayed and anxious. Together with the changing attitudes of some nurses, this has damaged relationships and resulted in both parties more carefully marking their territories. The new rules have also meant that it is more difficult to find systems that allow them to work as a team or new ways of working together to substitute the old established relationship (Fagin, 1992). Doctors, confused at the nurses' conduct, felt let down and uncomfortable, while nurses reacted with dismay to Stein's analysis. This alleged crisis in the doctor–nurse relationship, as with all crises, is transient, and at the beginning of the twenty-first century there are already signs that the relationship between doctors and nurses has developed further as technological and economic changes have caused radical changes in professional roles. Thus today it is extremely difficult to find supporters of Stain's earlier thesis. In addition, nurses should not be concerned, as the requirement on doctors to maintain their knowledge and technical expertise means that nurses play a key role in humanizing health care by maintaining a close relationship with patients. The professional relationship, given the present situation, especially in the hospital sector, can no longer be conceived in a unilateral manner, as other professionals must be involved in providing solutions to patients' problems. Finding resolutions of the interprofessional problems experienced by nurses and doctors is an ethical duty, and while the search continues it must be remembered that the patient – the reason for the existence of both professions and the ultimate objective of health care – must also be seen as a member of the relationship if attention and quality health care are to be offered, and if the trust which society has placed in the health professionals is to be deserved.

Studies on doctor–nurse relations

Considerable research into the doctor–nurse relationship has been undertaken. Most agree that the outdated conception of hierarchical relations, in which medical power could not be questioned, should be replaced by a conception involving collaboration. Within such collaborative working each professional would be responsible for an area and would provide particular elements of health care required by the population. Examples of such models include Alpert (1992), who developed a programme in the Beth Israel Hospital in Boston (USA) where doctors and nurses worked collaboratively in a specially designed unit. They defined this as something more than working closely together and as something more than doing their duty. The collaboration was an interaction, a union, of effort, which resulted in more than the sum of isolated activities. When the trial was completed they realized that their collaboration had also resulted in them taking full advantage of their different experiences and knowledge.

Baggs and Schmitt (1997) demonstrated that where doctors and nurses worked collaboratively and demonstrated mutual respect, patient care in intensive care improved, as did job satisfaction and cost control. Their collaborative working included being available, which involved being in the right place, having time and having appropriate knowledge, and being receptive, which involved being interested in each other.

Keen and Malby (1992), studying the effects of resource management in six NHS hospitals, showed that nurses did not always grasp the opportunity to enhance their power and practice. Fagin (1992) analysed the collaboration between doctors and nurses and demonstrated the existing advantages and disadvantages. She described the collaboration as a relationship of interdependence, which requires the recognition of complementary roles.

Arslanian-Engoren (1995), in a phenomenological qualitative study, tried to identify the experiences of clinical nurse specialists (CNS) and stressed the difficulties resulting from educational differences between doctors and nurses. She emphasized that if a working collaboration can be produced, this in turn creates a feeling of intense satisfaction among the professionals.

Porter (1991), through a participant observation study of power relations between nurses and doctors on an intensive care unit and a general medical ward, demonstrated that with the exception of the nurse–consultant interactions, nurses were less dependent on these subordinate modes of interaction than much of the literature suggested.

Makadon and Gibbons (1985) found similarities when 'sincere efforts will permit doctors and nurses to work together in a positive way in order to carry out the difficult task of providing high quality care at the lowest possible cost'. They believe that the reduced hospital stays, the increase in numbers of seriously ill patients in hospital and the decrease in resources create obligations of collaboration in management and expressed the view that the nurses' clinical competence and creativity could ease the doctors' work.

Prerequisites for successful interpersonal relationships

In all human relationships, and even more so among members of a team, specific prerequisites must be adhered to to help the relationship work and achieve the planned objectives.

Mutual respect

For many authors (Bayles, 1987; Baggs and Schmitt, 1997; McNair and Bryan, 1997), respect is a key element among team members. Respect must be considered from three perspectives. First, the other person must be respected as another human being with equal rights and with moral integrity. This naturally requires being polite and courteous, but it also means acknowledging their beliefs and values, and treating them as an equal. Even when someone's beliefs clash with our own, or their value system results in their inability to participate in certain procedures, such as assisting with a termination of pregnancy, their views must still be respected.

Second, team members must be respected as professionals. This means recognizing their legitimate area of responsibility and not interfering without extremely good grounds, such as patient safety. The grey areas where there are no clear lines of demarcation must be discussed by the team and agreement reached on who can intervene and where ultimate responsibility will lie. Doctors, nurses and other health professionals need to respect each other and recognize the different experience and knowledge that they bring to the team as a result of their work.

Third, there must be respect at a personal level, which involves accepting each other's individuality, personal capacities and limitations. This is of the utmost importance to achieve the patient's wellbeing, and a prerequisite for evaluating others is the need to evaluate oneself. In this way joint reflections on the effectiveness of the team can be undertaken in a non-judgemental atmosphere of mutual trust without fear of disparagement.

Communication and trust

Lack of communication is one of the principal problems found within health teams (Bayles, 1987; Fagin, 1992). Demanding workloads often mean that insufficient time is available for communication, and the working environment is often not conducive to sharing considerable amounts of sensitive information. Successful teamwork requires continuous clear, honest communication between team members and, although written agreements frequently mention this element of teamwork, it is often difficult to achieve in practice. Communication systems have been developed, time offered, training given and so on, but even these do not always achieve the objective. In reality, interpersonal communication is always a very complex process that requires certain attitudes of understanding, respect and veracity in all the participants.

Responsibility

A profession is not a skill, nor is it a simple occupation (Bayles, 1987; Gracia, 1998). This implies that with it come certain obligations. Gracia (1998) considers responsibility as a response, a 'realizing' or 'paying of dues', to oneself and to society, and that there exists, therefore, a personal, intimate level – one's conscious and another public level that is regulated by justice.

Being responsible is critical in interprofessional relationships, especially when faced with questions of professional incompetence. Both individual and collective responsibility exist in teamwork. The professional is not only responsible for his own actions, but also for patients receiving good quality health care from the team. This implies that when the professional is aware that a team member is not acting in an appropriate manner, an ethical dilemma arises in that the professional must decide whether or not to act. One difficulty in this type of situation is how any interference might affect the responsibilities of other team members. The problem becomes even greater when the situation involves a doctor and a nurse. For the welfare of the patient the responsibility of each team member must be clearly demarcated and defined. Under no circumstances can malpractice be tolerated, as the primary professional responsibility is for the patient's wellbeing.

Doctor–nurse relationships in Europe

Broadly speaking, nurses within the European Community find themselves in similar situations, with only slight differences found in their training and in the public health systems of each country. A university training where research and development in the science of nursing is guaranteed, as well as a national public health system, make equality among all health professionals much more of a reality.

Spain

Spanish nurses have undergone the same process of change in their activities and responsibilities, with the objective of obtaining recognition and attainment of their professional autonomy as nurses in other parts of Europe. This process was initiated rather later than in other European countries due to the political situation during the dictatorship, which did not facilitate the development of rights and liberties.

Following 1975, when democracy came into being, nurses were able to study at university but, more than two decades later, a degree in nursing has still not been recognized by the Ministry of Education and Science. This makes it even more difficult for nurses to attain certain levels of power and autonomy, and also impedes the development of the nursing science. The situation has resulted in nurses gaining degrees in other subjects, and recently, to embark on advanced nursing studies, which although not recognized by the Ministry, are awarded at degree level by the universities that run these programmes. It is hoped that in the not too distant future a degree in nursing will be fully recognized. In the field of education, relations between doctors and nurses pose other difficulties, which differ slightly from region to region. While in some regions nurses are recognized for their particular competencies, in others doctors still have the upper hand in terms of authority. Slowly, however, nurses' training is gradually improving, as is their autonomy and, as a consequence, they have gained credibility within universities.

In the hospital and primary care sectors, the situation is different. According to Gracia (1998), an analysis of the last twenty years does not reveal that the Spanish health system has undergone great changes. From the 1970s onwards, hospitals were characteristically well equipped and the charitable assistance on which many relied has been substituted by one based on obligatory contributions from citizens and the state. The state adopted a system similar to the national insurance system in the UK, the Obligatory Health Coverage (El Seguro Obligatorio de Enfermedad). This has stimulated entire sectors of the economy, such as the chemicals/pharmaceuticals industry, hospital installations and engineers to name but two; the consequences of this revolution have been spectacular, including:

1. A predominantly home based health service becoming hospital based.
2. A change in medical role from general family doctor to specialist as a natural consequence of the technological advances in diagnostic and therapeutic processes, which demand greater technical expertise in increasing areas of human pathology. (Gracia, 1998)

This process has also affected nursing, which has shadowed the changes in medicine by creating different specialities. Nurses also work in promoting health and preventing illness, and they have developed their responsibilities within their own area of knowledge. At present, both in primary and hospital care, nurses are gaining greater autonomy in their daily work, just as they are in education. Gradually their relationship with the doctors is changing as they are gaining greater recognition, and the most highly qualified among them are adopting strategies in which to develop their role.

Professional development of nurses has been hampered, however, by the economic crisis in health care, as this has demanded different methods of working and obliged professionals in all areas to redefine their areas of responsibility in order to utilize existing resources to the full. Some of these changes have been detrimental to the developing role of the nurse. Also, the widespread development and recognition of patients' rights has led to a greater focus on quality control, which in turn has placed additional burdens on all health professionals. Economic crisis together with drives for greater quality are producing confusion and may lead to demotivation, a reduction in self-esteem and staff 'burnout'.

Relations within the multi-diciplinary team benefit from the fact that the model for the Spanish health care system is universal and that private medicine is for a minority. This system allows all members of the team to be salaried, and to work under the same conditions, therefore sharing the same problems. Both nurses and doctors are concerned about interpersonal relations, and analysis of ethical codes for nursing emphasizes that the nurses' responsibilities are within the team, requiring relationships to be developed with other professionals, and especially other nurses. The doctors' code does not speak of their responsibilities within the team generally and makes no mention of their relationships with the nurses.

Some initiatives have been established to improve interprofessional relationships. Special groups analyse the origins of any conflicts and look for ways of resolving them. It is therefore worthwhile considering the role of ethical committees in teamworking. These committees enable thought and dialogue when multidisciplinary teams face ethical problems affecting the patient and various professionals. Conditions conducive to dialogue, such as meeting in a relaxed atmosphere, around a table, far from the hospital ward, enable problems to be discussed and analysed from an ethical perspective in which the ultimate interest of the deliberations is the patient rather than professional self-interest. This means that, gradually, team members have become mutually aware of each other's problems and can acknowledge similarities in their different viewpoints. Ethical committees are present in the majority of Spanish hospitals and primary care settings. The law ensures that the nurses are present both in clinical research and hospital committees and that they enjoy the same rights as all other members.

The United Kingdom (UK)

UK nurses have been pioneers in the development of nursing, and initiated processes for recognition of their autonomy some years ago. To study for a degree in nursing and continue through to postgraduate studies is not a problem in the UK, where suitably qualified nurses have every right to occupy university posts.

Both the hospitals and primary care sectors have been affected by the changes in the NHS. A study carried out by Keen and Malby (1992) demonstrated that the organizational changes which have taken place within the NHS since the 1980s ignored nurses, who consequently lost power and responsibility, and created confusion about their role in management and clinical practice. The study also indicated that the old 'doctor–nurse game' would have to be expanded to include three players – doctors, nurses and administrators – and that in the new version nurses have lost authority in management.

The UK Code of Professional Conduct (NMC, 2002) requires that nurses 'co-operate with others in the team'. It goes on to explain that this means the nurse is 'expected to work co-operatively within teams and to respect the skills, expertise and contributions of your colleagues. You must treat them fairly and without discrimination' (NMC, 2002, p. 6).

When this definition is applied to clinical practice there appear to be grey areas where problems exist in the doctor–nurse relationship. One problem frequently encountered is that nurses disagree with certain medical decisions and treatments, or with given orders. The emergence of specialist nurses has increased conflict between nurses and doctors concerning their respective areas of responsibility (Rumbold, 1999). These conflicts should be solved through dialogue and collaboration, rather than automatic submission on the part of nurses. As a professional, the nurse is morally responsible for her actions.

Conclusion

Technological advances and social changes within health systems of the European Community have had an enormous influence on doctor–patient relationships and have brought about many changes. The complex nature of knowledge required for effective health care today obliges health professionals to work as a team to solve the health problems facing modern societies. Throughout recent decades doctor–nurse collaboration has been considered as a major part of the solution to these problems. Although on an intellectual level, no one doubts that medicine and nursing are two autonomous professions that must work together for the wellbeing of the patient, the day-to-day reality is somewhat different. One or two decades are not sufficient, however, in spite of important changes that have taken place, such as nurse education moving into the university sector in many countries and nurses developing their own field of knowledge, for the traditional values of nursing's origin as a female occupation such as obedience and submissiveness to entirely disappear in such a short time.

Dialogue and collaboration are essential but for teamwork to really succeed each member of the team must embrace attitudes of respect, trust and responsibility towards each other as these qualities form the basis of any human relationship. It is only from this perspective that the health care team can be truly effective in promoting health, and preventing and curing illness.

References

Alpert, H.B., Goldman, L.D., Kilroy, C.M. and Pike, A.W. (1992) '7 Gryzmish: Toward an understanding of collaboration', *Nursing Clinics of North America*, **27** (1): 47–59.

Arroyo, M.P., Cortina, A., Torralba, M.J. and Zugasti, J. (1997) *Ética y Legislación en Enfermeria*, Madrid: McGraw-Hill Interamericana, pp. 51–58.

Arslanian-Engoren, C.M. (1995) 'Lived Experiences of CNSs Who Collaborate with Physicians: A Phenomenological Study', *Clinical Nurse Specialist*, **19** (2): 68–74.

Baggs, J.G. and Schmitt, M.H. (1997) 'Nurses and Resident Physicians' Perceptions of the Process of Collaboration in an MICU', *Research in Nursing & Health*, **20**: 71–80.

Bayles, M.D. (1987) 'Interprofessional Ethics in Health Care', *International Journal of Applied Philosophy*, **3**: 21–28.

Curtin, L. (1982) 'Autonomy, accountability and nursing practice', *Top Clin Nurs*, Apr, **4** (2): 7–14.

Curtin, L. and Flaherty, M.J. (1982) *Nursing Ethics, Theories and Pragmatics*, Englewood Cliffs, MD: Prentice-Hall International, pp. 137–151.

Fagin, C.M. (1992) 'Collaboration between Nurses and Physicians, no longer choice', *Nursing & Health Care*, **13**: 354–363.

Gracia, D. (1998) *Profesión médica, investigación y justicia sanitaria*, Bogota, DC: El Buho, pp. 32–57.

Jolley, M. and Allan, P. (eds) (1992) *Current Issues in Nursing*, London: Chapman & Hall, pp. 1–22.

Keen, J. and Malby, R. (1992) 'Nursing power and practice in the United Kingdom National Health Service', *Journal of Advanced Nursing*, **17**: 863–870.

Makadon, H.J. and Gibbons, M.P. (1985) 'Nurses and physicians: prospects for collaboration', *Ann Intern Med*, Jul, **103** (1): 134–136.

McNair, S.M. and Bryan, G.W. (1997) 'The Physician–Nurse Relationship in Family Practice', *The Canadian Nurse (L'Infirmière Canadienne)*, August: 31–33.

NMC (Nursing and Midwifery Council) (2002) *Code of Professional Conduct*, London: NMC.

Porter, S. (1991) 'A participant observation study of power relations between nurses and doctors in a general hospital', *Journal of Advanced Nursing*, **16**: 728–735.

Rumbold, G. (1999) *Ethics in Nursing Practice*, 3rd edn, London: Baillière Tindall, pp. 177–199.

Stein, L.L. (1967) 'The doctor–nurse game', *Arch Gen Psychiatry*, Jun, **16** (6): 699–703.

Stein, L.L. Watts, D.T. and Howell, T. (1990) 'The doctor–nurse game revised', *New England Journal of Medicine*, **322** (8): 546–549.

7

The Nurse: Autonomous Professional or Subservient Worker?

P. Anne Scott

Introduction

> about the only features held constant from one author to another are that
> autonomy is a feature of persons and that it is a desirable quality to have.
>
> (Dworkin, 1988, p. 6)

Autonomy is a concept frequently met with in the literature on professional nursing practice, professional ethics and health care ethics. Ideas regarding the meaning of the concept are wide and varied. Etymologically the word comes from the Greek: *autos* (self) and *nomos* (rule or law). It appears that the term was first applied to the Greek city-states, to describe a state of self-rule or independence, in the political sense. This notion of 'self-rule', or 'independence' or 'self-determination' is at least part of what seems to be commonly understood in contemporary uses of the concept. However, some authors, for example, Young (1986) draw attention to an important distinction between the notion of 'self-rule' or 'independence' and 'self-determination', which may be being overlooked by some theorists.

Young suggests that failure to attend to this distinction may lead one to focus almost exclusively on the Millean idea of negative liberty, which is freedom to do as one wants so long as it does not interfere with or harm others, and on external constraints on the agent's autonomy. This focus neglects the positive, proactive elements in individual autonomy or the self-determining ability to author one's own life. It also excludes a consideration of internal constraints on autonomy such as irrational or non-rational impulses and drives which derives from a Kantian approach to the autonomy issue. A shift of focus to encompass the positive, proactive, self-determining elements in individual autonomy, and to consider the influence of the internal constraints on autonomy is worth while when attempting to clarify the nature of, and the constraints upon, autonomy within a nursing context.

It may be argued, for example, that the autonomous practice of the nurse is seriously curtailed at certain points during clinical practice. For example, even though he or she knows that Mr Smith needs a bronchial dilating drug prescribed urgently, the nurse must wait either until a doctor voluntarily realizes this and prescribes the required drug or until the doctor is successfully cajoled, by the nurse, into doing so. A case similar to this is discussed by Benner, Tanner and Chesla (1996, pp. 281–283). Another example relates to the notion of whistle-blowing. It is suggested that many nurses do not blow the whistle on malpractice or neglect because, rather than supporting the nurse's concern for patients and relatives in such a case, the hospital hierarchy and administration may make the particular nurse's life unbearable, or dismiss the nurse from employment (Corea, 1977, p. 65; Hunt, 1995, p. 16).

While such situations undoubtedly do occur, whether they are examples of interference with the nurse's autonomy is another matter. This type of issue will be discussed further below.

Summary

To aid the discussion a number of the elements surrounding autonomy need to be clarified. The first of these to be explored is the relationship between autonomy and freedom; in particular, notions of coercion and responsibility are examined. Next the question as to whether autonomy is a right or an aspect of character is addressed, before we examine the notion of moral autonomy. It is here that the concepts of accountability, responsibility and authority are considered, together with their relationship to autonomy.

The chapter then addresses the question of whether an individual can ever be fully autonomous, and considers what an individual's autonomy interests might be. Finally the chapter addresses the issue of autonomy and the nurse, and particularly what is required by professional autonomy and professional responsibility.

Autonomy and freedom

Perhaps one of the first things to consider is the relationship between freedom and autonomy. It is evident that autonomy should not be seen as synonymous with freedom. Many animals may be free to run around as they wish, to feed as they wish, but they are not considered to be autonomous beings. Very young children in many societies are free from the rigours of work or the demands of citizenship; however, they also are not considered autonomous beings. Freedom therefore can not be said to be a sufficient condition for autonomy to exist. Is freedom, then, even a necessary condition for the ascription of autonomy?

At first glance it would seem reasonable to suggest that to be autonomous, a person must have at least some degree of freedom. However, to say that freedom (in the above sense of no external restrictions) is important on many occasions for the exercise of autonomy is not the same as saying that such freedom is a necessary condition for autonomy to exist.

A notion closely linked with autonomy is responsibility. A consequence of autonomous action is that the autonomous agent is thereby responsible for that action. If one can be held responsible for one's actions under coercion, or while following orders, then it is possible to argue, with Dworkin (1988), that freedom is not even a necessary condition for autonomy to exist. The question therefore is, 'Can one legitimately be held responsible for one's actions when these actions are carried out "under orders" or under duress?'

It seems that to answer this question a number of different issues need to be taken into account. First, it seems important to recognize the impact of context. During periods of political unrest and terrorist activity the following scenario is a realistic possibility. Armed terrorists are holding a gun to the head of your spouse or child. They demand that you drive a car containing a large bomb to a busy shopping area and park the car outside a well-known department store. There is good reason to believe that your loved one will be murdered if the demands of the terrorists are not met. You face a serious dilemma here. In choosing the life of your family over the lives of main-street shoppers, and delivering the terrorist bomb as ordered, your actions are made completely comprehensible by the context. If your actions are not condoned in this situation, they are not normally condemned either. None the less your decision in this horrific situation is still your own decision and therefore your responsibility.

Second, in situations of coercion, or the carrying out of orders, the notion of role enactment seems to be of relevance (Downie, 1964; Scott, 1997). Role enactment refers to those qualities that an individual brings to his or her role. These qualities are elements of the character and are thus not reducible to aspects of the role.

Bettelheim (1960) describes how various inmates in the Nazis' concentration camps reacted to being given varying degrees of authority over other inmates. He identified the Jehovah's Witnesses as the group who, although following orders, still retained a humane attitude toward their fellow inmates over whom they were placed in authority by the German forces. Unlike many other groups in a similar position, the Jehovah's Witnesses did not begin to identify with the repressive regime.

It may be the case that in some situations of coercion or 'following orders' the quality of one's role enactment is all that is under one's control. For example, in the case cited by Bettelheim, none of the prisoners, including those raised to positions of authority over others, had any power to increase rations or improve the external resources for the care of the sick or starving, or change work orders. Those in positions of some authority could, however, make various situations easier for the less well-off prisoners under their charge. Those in authority could show the other prisoners humanity in various restricted ways. The Jehovah's Witnesses did this consistently as a group. They did not use their position of power to oppress others when they gained the power to do so, despite having been victims of such oppression themselves.

What one does is important, but so also is the manner in which one does it. In some situations, such as that described above, one may feel obliged to do certain tasks as a result of coercion. In these situations what one does may no longer be under one's direct control. However, despite this external restriction on one's autonomy, one may retain control over the manner in which one does the particular task. An example from clinical practice will perhaps elucidate the point here. I may know or be told that a patient needs two-hourly turning to prevent pressure problems. I therefore turn the patient every two hours. However, the manner in which I turn the patient usually makes a difference to the patient. This is especially likely to be the case if, for example, she or he is suffering post-operative discomfort or arthritic pain. However, if the manner or quality of enactment can be separated from the task or role, then the manner of enactment is a direct and significant moral responsibility as, of course, is one's decision to submit to coercion or orders rather than face the consequences of failing to do this.

Certain situations cannot sensibly be seen to warrant such drastic action as risking unemployment, even if the agent does not think that the other options are particularly good ones in the moral sense. The decision being reached is based on the individual's value judgements and in this sense the individual is making an autonomous decision. The weighing of the options, together with the decision taken, is the responsibility of the moral agent involved.

This leads one to conclude that freedom of *action*, in the sense of overt observable behaviour, is not a necessary condition for autonomy to exist, whereas freedom of thought, in the sense of having the intellectual apparatus and psychological freedom, may well be a necessary condition. It appears to be freedom in the direct *freedom of action* sense that Dworkin intends in the following:

> Freedom is neither necessary nor sufficient for autonomy. Not only are they different concepts, their scope is different. Freedom is a local concept; autonomy is a global one. The question of freedom is decided at specific points in time. He was free to do such and such at a particular time. At a later date he was not free to do that. Whereas questions of autonomy can only be assessed over extended portions of a person's life. It is a dimension of assessment that evaluates a whole way of living one's life. (Dworkin, 1988, p. 60)

Autonomy – a right or an aspect of character?

Given that it is possible to argue, as Dworkin (1988) does, that autonomy is something that can be assessed by looking at an extended portion of a person's life, two further points of interest arise. First, is autonomy a right to which at least certain people have claims, or is autonomy a quality of personhood or character? The answer to this question is likely to have important implications for the notion that there are internal as well as external constraints on autonomy.

Some health care ethics literature seems to imply that autonomy is a right to which certain people have a legitimate claim. This implication may be seen in references to the right to self-determination (for example Valimaki, Leino-Kilpi and Helenius, 1996). However, foetuses, children, the mentally handicapped, the mentally ill and the senile are not considered to have a valid claim to the right to be autonomous – or their right to be recognized as autonomous is restricted in important ways. One may therefore begin to move closer to the idea that autonomy is more accurately linked with certain human characteristics or aspects of human development than an externally regulated entity such as a right to which one is entitled. Thomasma (1995) argues that 'Speaking descriptively, autonomy can be viewed as a feature of individual identity and integrity.'

An individual may lay claim to the right to exercise his or her autonomy, but this is a different issue. Mrs Jones may be considered an autonomous person, who in certain situations is enabled to exercise her autonomy, while in other situations she cannot do so. Analogously, Mrs Jones may be considered a sensitive individual. In a certain role Mrs Jones may feel that she cannot, or is not being enabled to, show her sensitivity in the manner or to the extent that she might wish.

The idea that autonomy is a personal characteristic or quality echoes Dworkin's suggestion that autonomy is a global concept, the existence of which can only accurately be assessed over time. A personal characteristic or quality is multidimensional. It is capable of being formed, developed, sustained or thwarted, diminished or destroyed by the working of internal and/or external factors.

On the other hand a right lacks this degree of complexity. The practically important aspect of a right is external to the person; that is, the right is either granted or withheld. One can sensibly speak of degrees of autonomy as one can speak of degrees of creative ability or intelligence. It does not seem immediately evident that it is sensible to speak of degrees of a right. Either one has a right to get married, practise law or medicine, drive a car, get a divorce, or practise certain religious rituals, or one does not have such a right. What would it mean to state that a particular individual had any of these rights to a certain degree?

Working on the assumption that autonomy is a characteristic or a quality of a person, acceptance of the idea that there are internal as well as external constraints on autonomy would seem to be fairly straightforward. The commonly accepted stance that certain groups of human beings (as well as lower animals) are incapable of autonomous action, choice, or decision is supportive of the idea that there are internal constraints on personal autonomy. Children are a case in point. Children below a certain age are often deemed to lack the minimum degree of emotional, psychological, physical and/or intellectual maturity required for the exercise of personal autonomy. This is the case for a variety of decisions, actions or commitments. The behaviour of a young child is still too strongly influenced by drives and impulses.

The psychological, emotional, intellectual and physical development of an individual, that is, the factors internal to the individual, are crucial to the development of an individual's autonomy. These factors are at least as significant to individual autonomy as are external factors such as social structures or other persons.

Moral autonomy

A pertinent question to pose here is: 'Is moral autonomy a subset of the general concept of autonomy or is moral autonomy an entirely separate entity?' Young (1986, p. 49) suggests that

> An autonomous life is one that is directed in accordance with an individual's own conception of what he (or she) wants to do in and with that life. Such an account requires us to think of autonomy as involving more than just the absence of constraints. A purely 'negative' conception (absence of constraints) leaves out the positive element of self-determination essential to an adequate account of autonomy.

The idea of living life according to one's own conception of what one wants to do in and with that life seems to suggest that the concept of autonomy is substantively empty. Should this worry us?

Society is made up of individuals with a vast number of different social roles, aspirations and priorities. My responsibilities, aspirations and priorities are part of me and my life just as your aspirations, priorities and responsibilities are of you and your life. It does not seem possible to argue that our various responsibilities, aspirations or priorities should or even could be the same. Yet each of us may have, and frequently exercise, a relatively high degree of personal autonomy. It would seem, therefore, that the concept of autonomy is, of necessity, substantively empty. What is not immediately evident is exactly why this should be considered a problem with the concept.

One cannot define an autonomous individual as an individual who lives life according to his or her own particular lights, and takes responsibility for this, while at the same time wanting to state substantively what decisions or actions autonomous decisions or actions are. This, of course, is not to adopt a crudely relativistic stance and say that any decision or action is as good as any other. It is, however, to say that an autonomous decision or action, made by person X, is a decision or action which X performs or reaches via his or her own reflective processes. Such a decision or action is not reached or performed under such influences as brainwashing, manipulation or blind faith.

It is at least something like the above process that gives rise to, or is indicative of, the quality of autonomy in an individual. It seems, therefore, that moral autonomy is a subset of general personal autonomy, rather than something completely separate. Moral autonomy can reasonably be assumed to include the making of considered moral choices. These choices are made following reflection on what the individual understands as good and bad, right and wrong. These choices are made within the context of an attempt to live life according to one's own conception of what one wants to do in and with that life. This is not to take the individual out of his or her social context and to see the living of a life as a purely individualistic or even selfish process. But it is to place the onus on the individual person to weigh up and deal with the mutual interaction and responsibilities of the self, with family, friends, community and society.

A short digression seems opportune here. One may wish to argue that issues of individual responsibility and the implication of mutual interaction and dependence are not particularly well aired in nursing literature or policy. The irony of this suggestion is evident once one considers the UKCC Code of Professional Conduct (1992), for example. This code seemed to place the entire responsibility for the delivery of decent nursing care on the shoulders of the individual practitioner. In fact the code has been criticized frequently for this. Thus the then regulatory body in the UK clearly articulated that the individual nurse is professionally responsible for his or her actions and provided guidance on the interpretation of what this might mean (UKCC, 1996). This position is similalrly reflected in the latest Code of Professional Conduct published by the Nursing and Midwifery Council (2002).

An Bord Altranais has followed a similar line in Southern Ireland (An Bord Altranais, 1988) and is currently showing signs of strengthening the profession's teeth in terms of tightening up on the importance of their code of practice (Government of Ireland, 1998). The problem appears to be in the collective interpretation of the nursing profession of what this demand on the individual practitioner actually means.

Perhaps one of the basic problems is that those who strongly influence the shape and development of codes of practice for nurses have worked with implicit assumptions of relatively strong levels of collegiality and peer review, which in fact only exists in embryonic form in many clinical nursing contexts. As indicated in the above discussion of autonomy, one does not exist in isolation. This is as true for the individual nurse as it is for the lay person. If the structure and organization of the nurse's clinical environment is outside the individual practitioner's control, then demanding that the practitioner be fully accountable for their practice is either a totally unrealistic demand or naïve in the extreme. It may also lead to high levels of moral distress in practitioners. This issue was clearly recognized by the recent Commission on Nursing in the South of Ireland. The Commission reports:

> A range of issues was raised during the consultative process in relation to the role of nurses and midwives in the management of services. These concerns included the need for greater internal communication within organisations, a need for the greater involvement of nurses and midwives in planning and policy development, a concern that nursing and midwifery management was preoccupied with hierarchies and the detailed control of nurses and midwives, rather than the management of the professional function and the related need for the greater devolution of authority within the nursing and midwifery management structure. (Government of Ireland, 1998, p. 5)

The Commission goes on to state that

> Structural reforms within nursing and midwifery management are required. There needs to be greater devolution of authority to nursing and midwifery management at the unit of care level. Senior nursing and midwifery management should focus to a much greater extent on strategic planning and quality assurance. Middle nursing management needs to be given clearly delegated responsibility such as in the management of an area of care or designated functional responsibilities. The Commission considers first line nursing as essential to the effective operation and on-going development of a high quality service. First line nursing and midwifery managers have to balance management skills with clinical credibility. (Ibid.)

In a very pertinent analysis of the issues of work organization and professional autonomy in the UK, Duff (1995, p. 54) suggests that 'The principal consequence of autonomy is accountability'. By this Duff means being answerable for one's actions. She points out that in, for example, the junior doctor–consultant relationship, the junior doctor is not fully autonomous. She or he is only autonomous within the defined parameters of their expertise. The junior doctor is accountable for the care given and the clinical decisions reached. But the consultant is also 'partially accountable through the exercise of their supervisory function'.

Duff goes on to suggest that primary nursing provides an example of how a similar system of work organization, namely one that is collegial and based on peer review, can work in nursing. However, she also points out that the traditional hierarchical accountability system is still alive and well within the contexts in which many nurses practice. This seems to be particularly the case in institution-based practice settings.

> There is only a limited sense in which a nurse can, in any way, be said to be accountable for the discharge of responsibilities based on a plan of action and protocols decided by someone else. The nurse lacks the necessary authority and autonomy. (Duff, 1995, p. 54)

As the report from the Irish Commission, quoted above, indicates, this refers to nursing management and organizational style just as much, if not more, than it does to medical prescriptions of clinical care.

A study carried out by Michael Bowman also seems pertinent here. Bowman's exploratory study considered the role of the registered nurse and was conducted in two district health authorities in the UK.

> Nurses perceive the core of the problem to be their workload, with too much to do and too few resources, together with the inordinate pressures of coping with change, organisational and technological; in addition there are the ever increasing demands of informed patients on matters relating to their health, care and progress, with rights enshrined in the Patient's Charter (DHSS 1991) and 'Statements of Intent' delivered by some health authorities and hospital trusts. Ward sisters and staff nurses commented:

> 'We have the responsibility and accountability to ensure resources, but no authority to enable their acquisition' and 'It is difficult to ensure high standards of care without having control over resources, staffing and materials'. Nurse managers stated that it was their function to initiate and regulate ward resources; nurses were not involved beyond the requisition stage. (Bowman, 1995, p. 1)

Issues of authority, responsibility and accountability are intimately linked with the concept of autonomy. I can do no more in this short chapter but draw attention to this fact and to urge the nursing profession and our leaders to spend time and effort considering these issues and their implication for future configurations and organization of nursing work. However, what the above quote indicates is that nurses themselves, sometimes in the guise of nurse managers, may be constraining the professional autonomy of their nursing colleagues and peers just as much if not more than our colleagues in the medical profession.

A further issue that needs to be addressed within this context is the apparent 'blind spot' that nurses, *en masse*, seem to develop – possibly as a side effect of professional socialization. This 'blind spot' may spring from the human tendency to generalize from one incident. Such a tendency is recognized in the health promotion literature, when for example the smoker, attempting to stop, has one cigarette. Instead of interpreting this as one slip, the individual has a second and third cigarette and so on, perceiving the first slip as indicative of such weakness of will as to make reform impossible.

It seems that nurses have a similar tendency to generalize from one area of curtailed or lack of autonomy to perceive their entire practice, and practice context, to be beyond their control. Bowman (1995) draws attention to the perceived lack of autonomy by ward sisters and/or staff nurses which need not be an accurate perception and which, in the eyes of some, was not in fact an accurate perception of the situation.

> The officers of the statutory and professional bodies generally perceived the non-use of the authority and autonomy by some professional nurses, which could be attributed to traditional reasons, i.e. nurses' perceived subordinate role to other professionals, coupled with nurses' lack of assertiveness and their inability to make decisions, as substantially contributing to nurses inability to meet their statutory obligations. (Bowman, 1996, p. 57)

Perhaps Chadwick and Tadd (1992, p. 57) provide some focus to this analysis when they state:

> Nurses often fail to recognise that because they form the interface between patients, their relatives and doctors, they are in fact very powerful. By educating patients and their relatives to ask pertinent questions, this power could effectively transferred to the patient enabling him and his relatives to obtain relevant information.

They continue:

> Nurses must be aware of reducing ethical decisions to either clinical or medical ones and of claiming to be powerless in an attempt to avoid shouldering one's moral responsibilities. (Ibid.)

I suggest that the above discussion provides some evidence of a lack of insight by nurses into how the profession's traditional allegiance and perpetuation of line management potentially stymies nurses' abilities to be autonomous professionals and to exercise individual professional and moral responsibility. An argument in support of the accuracy of this claim can be found in Scott (1998). Yet ironically a lot of scholarship regarding the nature of nursing emphasizes the inherently moral nature of the nursing endeavour (Bishop and Scudder, 1990; Chadwick and Tadd, 1992; Gastmans *et al.*, 1998). Therefore this is an issue deserving further thought and exploration.

However, to return from our digression: at this point it is being argued that autonomy is:

- not synonymous with freedom of action or independence;
- a quality of a person rather than a right to which one lays claim;
- influenced by internal as well as by external constraints.

It is also suggested that in discussing autonomy one should take cognizance of the fact that people exist in a social milieu. Any account of autonomy should take this feature of human existence into account.

Can one be fully autonomous?

The notion that human beings are reproduced and survive in a social context or network would seem to have important implications for the possibility of anyone being fully autonomous. Empirical research in the areas of developmental psychology and sociology strongly suggests that the growing individual is crucially influenced by the views, attitudes and values of the family or community within which he or she develops.

Many of these influences are seen to endure throughout the person's life, and there are a number of examples in the literature:

- Individuals subjected to violence and battering during childhood seem to be at higher risk of battering their own children should they achieve parenthood (Gelles, 1997).
- Women whose mothers were battered by their husbands or partners are prone to choose potentially violent partners or spouses and to accept violence from them for lengthy periods of time before seeking

outside help (Gelles, 1997; Renvoize, 1978; Egger and Crancher, 1982).

- Girls reared in polygamous cultures, which have little contact with other societies, are more likely to accept polygamous marriages willingly than are girls from Western societies. Similarly for arranged marriages.

It seems, therefore, that in terms of living one's life and identifying one's values and priorities, an individual does not begin with a *tabula rasa*. Indeed, it is probably one of the greatest survival advantages of human existence that each individual does not constantly have to reinvent the wheel, as it were. However, this does call into question the notion of any individual having the potential to be totally autonomous. Thomasma (1995) and Downie and Telfer (1971) in fact dismiss the possibility as being incompatible with the social contexts within which human beings generally live and grow.

Autonomy interests

Lindley (1986, p. 181) suggests that

> There are two sorts of interest in autonomy – interests in its development and maintenance, and in its exercise. A person's autonomy interests may be harmed either by limiting her capacity for autonomy, or by preventing its exercise.

This seems an important distinction to draw and it does mirror the notion of autonomy being affected by internal and external factors. Although the development, maintenance and exercise of autonomy are likely to be affected by an interaction of internal and external constraints, internal constraints may have more of an influence on the development and maintenance of autonomy and external constraints on the exercise of autonomy. For example, imagine that one's psycho-social experiences over a prolonged period of time nudge one in the direction of developing fairly strong dependence and submissive characteristics or qualities. This experience would seem to militate against even the most liberal organizational structures in the workplace, resulting in one displaying much autonomous action or thought.

As was suggested earlier, autonomy is not an all-or-nothing affair. It will exist to varying degrees in different people. It does seem possible to suggest, however, that given a certain minimal level of intellectual and emotional maturity people can be helped towards autonomy. For example, in family life children may be given increasing responsibilities for certain tasks, for themselves and for others, perhaps younger siblings. Responsibilities may be increased with the child's age and experience. This is also in fact how many of us attempt to work with newly qualified or junior staff – as the Duff example, cited above, indicates.

Exercise of autonomy maintains a sense of personal autonomy and the ability to be autonomous, over time. The effect of persistent prohibition on the exercise of autonomy by the individual, even for a relatively limited period, is likely to be dramatic, as is evidenced by the results of empirical studies such as those on learned helplessness by Seligman in the 1970s.

Autonomy and the nurse

In the health care setting one is presented with a microcosm within which to consider autonomy, as against the macrocosm of general social existence. For example, the idea that personal autonomy is not synonymous with freedom of action or simple independence seems as applicable in the health care setting as in the wider social context. The notion that there are external and internal constraints on the development and maintenance of autonomy on the one hand, and on the exercise of autonomy on the other, seems as true for the health care setting as for other areas of human existence. For example, employment contracts, occupational hierarchies, multiple demands on the practitioner's loyalty and often multiple obligations are some of the more obvious external constraints on the autonomy of the nurse. Interestingly, it is suggested that nurses are more often victims of external constraints on their autonomy than are doctors (Hunt, 1994).

It may be argued, for instance, that whereas doctors are autonomous practitioners responsible only to their patients, nurses are responsible not only to their patients but also to their line managers and to their employers. This argument, however, does seem indicative of at least a degree of perceptual inertia. In most societies with organized systems of health care this is not an accurate description of the situation – except perhaps for the limited number of doctors who own their own hospitals or work solely in private practice, although even then there is normally some form of external authority.

In health care institutions such as hospitals, doctors as well as nurses are subject to the hierarchical structures of their professional organization and to the resource constraints imposed by their employers. As indicated above, however, Duff (1995) makes an interesting comment regarding how the hierarchical medical structures are managed. Duff's argument regarding the potential value of collegiality and review versus external control and punishment is worthy of some thought by practising nurses and senior members of our profession. It is to be hoped that the Report of the Commission on Nursing cited above should force some serious thought on this issue in the South of Ireland over the next few years.

An incident is described briefly at the beginning of this chapter regarding a nurse who knows the appropriate medication for a patient, but is either overruled by a doctor, or has to wait and/or cajole one into prescribing the medication. Such cases are cited in the literature as evidence of the subordination of the nurse, or of restrictions on his or her professional autonomy. There are a number of issues involved in this type of case.

First, and perhaps least importantly, it seems necessary to consider the role and the job description of the nurse. Even though this may be reasonably clear, at least in general terms, it will vary with the work situation in which the nurse finds herself. In many health care institutions and contexts in the UK, Ireland, Finland and USA, for example, prescription of drugs is not within the remit of the nurse (nurse practitioner roles and nurse prescribing programmes in the UK excepted). However, prescription of certain drugs is within the job description of community nurses working in rural Kenya for example, as it is within the clinical remit of the midwife.

It is possible to argue that the nurse is exercising personal autonomy in accepting a nursing post with whatever restrictions or extended role responsibilities the job involves. Perhaps such acceptance can be likened to the Roman Catholic priest's acceptance of the vow of obedience, or a priest as a member of a religious order taking a vow of poverty. Having accepted the limits of one's role from the outset it then becomes incumbent on the individual professional to work with colleagues to test the limits as perceived and to encourage, support and/or drive change where appropriate grounds exist for doing so. This, I suggest, is an aspect of professional responsibility and a manifestation of professional autonomy.

Second, if an inexperienced doctor overrides the considered suggestion of a nurse, then the nurse has at least two options. The nurse may either:

- determine that the patient is not going to be harmed in any significant way, and therefore decide to 'bite' his or her tongue; or,
- following reasonable attempts to get an explanation for the doctor's decision, states that he or she is not happy with the situation and is therefore going to seek further advice from the medical team involved.

Certainly a degree of diplomacy may be needed in this type of situation; however, it does seem that unnecessary conflict can be prevented by good communication skills. The focus of concern here should be the patient. If the patient, in the eyes of the nurse, is likely to be harmed by the doctor's decision, then the nurse has both a professional and a moral responsibility to take the matter further. This seems entirely clear from the codes of practice in UK, Ireland and Finland, for example.

Finally, I suggest that in our literature there is a tendency to confuse autonomous practice with moral autonomy. For example, many nurses, perhaps most in western societies, are not fully autonomous practitioners. Either by definition, or evolution of practice roles, part of the nurse's work is dependent on medical decisions and prescription. In so far as this is the case, nurses cannot be fully autonomous in their practice. The institutional structures within which nurses work and professional organizations, for example via codes of practice, perpetuate this link as appropriate. These latter two constraints, institutional structures and professional organizations, also affect the potential for autonomous practice by doctors.

However, from a nursing perspective at least two issues are significant here:

1. The extent to which the nurse's work is dependent on medical decision and prescription varies with the work context. In most European countries it seems to be the case that nurses working in the acute care sector will have more of their practices influenced and shaped by the medical and indeed the paramedical professions

than colleagues who are in community or consultancy practice. This is because the acute care sector is dominated by high-tech medical approaches to diagnosis and treatment. However, with the growth of specialist practitioner roles in the UK, for example, and the recommended development of these posts and those of advanced practitioner in Southern Ireland, there is an increasing degree of variation in the ability of the individual nurse to increase the degree of autonomous practice even for nurses within the acute care sector.

2. Given that the work of most, if not all, nurses is determined by medical need – at least to some degree – it is not the case that all the activities of nurses are so determined. There are many aspects of nursing practice that are directly under nursing control, for example, how hospital wards are managed, how caseloads are managed, how individual interactions with patients are managed. The question, of course, is how do nurses manage this aspect of their role and, particularly, are nurses potentially their own worst enemies here? Bowman (1995) seems especially relevant here and provides some grounds for suggesting a positive response to the question.

Conclusion

As suggested above, full personal autonomy is an unlikely possibility for any human being. It would seem that, in like manner, given the current context of health care practice, full professional autonomy is also not possible. If, as suggested above, health care practice is seen as a microcosm of wider society, then professional autonomy, like moral autonomy, can be seen as a subset of personal autonomy. However, it is clear that professional autonomy is not the same thing as moral autonomy. It also appears that nurses have some way to go, in terms of professional maturity, before it can confidently be claimed that they are autonomous professionals.

References

An Bord Altranais (1988) *The Code of Professional Conduct for each Nurse and Midwife*, Dublin: An Bord Altranais.

Benner, P., Tanner, C.A. and Chesla, C.A. (1996) *Expertise in Nursing Practice: Caring, Clinical Judgement and Ethics*, New York, NY: Springer Publishing Co.
Bettelheim, B. (1960) *The Informed Heart: The Human Condition in Modern Mass Society*, Illinois: The Free Press of Glencoe.
Bishop, A.H. and Scudder, J.R. (1990) *The Practical, Moral and Personal Sense of Nursing: A Phenomenological Philosophy of Practice*, New York: State University Press.
Bowman, M. (1995) *The Professional Nurse Coping with Change Now and in the Future*, London: Chapman Hall.
Bowman, M. (1996) *The professional nurse*, London: Chapman and Hall.
Chadwick, R. and Tadd, W. (1992) *Ethics Nursing and Practice: A Case Study Approach*, Basingstoke: Macmillan Education.
Corea, G. (1977) *The Hidden Malpractice: How American Medicine Treats Women as Patients and Professionals*, New York: William Morrow.
Downie, R.S. (1964) *Government Action and Morality*, London: Macmillan.
Downie, R.S. and Telfer, E. (1971) 'Autonomy', *Philosophy*, **156**: 293–301.
Dworkin, G. (1988) *The Theory and Practice of Autonomy*, New York: Cambridge University Press.
Duff, L. (1995) 'Standards of care, quality assurance and accountability', in Watson, R. (ed.) *Accountability in nursing practice*, London: Chapman and Hall, pp. 49–69.
Egger, S.J. and Crancher, J. (1982) 'Wife battering: an analysis of the victim's point of view', *Australian Family Physician*, **11**: 830–832.
Gastmans, C. Dierckx de Casterle and Schotsmans, P. (1998) 'Nursing considered as Moral practice: A Philosophical–Ethical Interpretation of Nursing', *Kennedy Institute of Ethics Journal*, **8**: 43–68.
Gelles, R.J. (1997) *Intimate Violence in Families*, 3rd edn, Thousand Oaks, CA: Sage.
Government of Ireland (1998) *Report of The Commission on Nursing. A Blueprint for the Future*, Dublin: Stationery Office.
Hunt, G. (1994) (ed.) *Ethical Issues in Nursing*, London: Routledge.
Hunt, G. (ed.) (1995) *Whistleblowing in the Health Service: Accountability, Law and Professional Practice*, London: Edward Arnold.
Lindley, R. (1986) *Autonomy*, London: Macmillan.
Mill, J.S. (1974) *On Liberty*, Harmondsworth, Middlesex: Penguin Group.
Nursing and Midwifery Council (2002) *Code of Professional Conduct*, London: NMC.
Renvoize, J. (1978) *Web of Violence: A Study of family Violence*, Harmondsworth, Middlesex: Pelican Books.
Scott, P.A. (1997) 'Imagination in Practice', *Journal of Medical Ethics*, **23**: 45–50.
Scott, P.A. (1998) 'Professional ethics: Are We on the Wrong Track?', *Nursing Ethics*, **5**: 477–485.

Seligman, M.E.P. (1975) *Helplessness: On Depression, Development and Death*, Reading: Freeman.
Thomasma, D.C. (1995) 'Beyond Autonomy to the Person Coping With Illness', *Cambridge Quarterly of Health Care Ethics*, **4**: 12–22.
United Kingdom Central Council for Nursing, Midwifery and Health Visiting (1992) *Code of Professional Conduct*, London: UKCC.
United Kingdom Central Council for Nursing, Midwifery and Health Visiting (1996) *Guidelines for Professional Practice*, London: UKCC.
Valimaki, M., Leino-Kilpi, H. and Helenius, H. (1996) 'Self-determination in Clinical Practice: the Psychiatric Patient's Point of View', *Nursing Ethics*, **3**: 329–344.
Young, R. (1986) *Personal Autonomy: Beyond Negative Belief and Positive Liberty*, London: Croom Helm.

8

Do Nurses have a Special Claim to be Patient Advocates?

Peter Allmark

Introduction

While many nurses claim to be patients' advocates, others see the role as impossible or undesirable for nurses. Although the advocacy movement has been strongest in northern Europe, similar movements are springing up in some southern European countries. It is important, therefore, that nurses across Europe consider fully the pros and cons of adopting the role of advocate. This chapter is concerned with the controversies surrounding advocacy and after a thorough discussion of the issues, it suggests some potential resolutions.

Summary

First, the history of advocacy and the emergence of the problem is explored. Following this, it is suggested that the key problem is that while there is agreement that the advocate will plead the patient's cause, there is disagreement over what that cause is. Three broad types of cause seem to emerge: rights, interest and autonomy. There are two problems with these types.

The first problem to be examined is that the terms themselves are internally ambiguous, so that it is not obvious what the advocate for someone's interest will plead. None the less it is suggested that nurses can fulfil the role of advocate for some of these categories. On the other hand it is doubtful that nurses have any special claim to be an advocate of any type. The second problem is that many definitions of advocacy conflate more than one type, and these types may conflict. Thus the advocate may find herself having to plead opposing causes. The next section attempts to show how the understanding that has emerged can resolve the problem with which we began. Those supporting advocacy usually have in mind the advocacy nurses can perform, especially in protecting the patient's legal rights. Those opposed have in mind the advocacy nurses cannot perform, especially in supporting the patient's autonomous choices. The question of whether it is possible to resolve the dispute between the two sides is then raised and three possible resolutions are considered.

History of advocacy and its associated problems

There seem to be two separate, though related, histories in the development of the problem: (1) independent advocacy, and (2) nursing advocacy.

Independent advocacy

The seeds of independent advocacy were sown in the civil rights era of the late 1960s, particularly in the USA (Brendon, 1991, pp. 119–123) although there had been concerns about the neglect of the rights of psychiatric patients since at least the early 1950s. In 1968 a New York civil liberties organization launched a national project aimed at protecting and expanding the rights of such patients. This mainly involved legal action on behalf of inmates and patients of different mental health institutions and one of those involved was Larry Gostin. Gostin forged papers to get himself admitted as a patient/inmate of a secure psychiatric hospital in North Carolina. He saw many abuses and, on his release, launched a series of successful lawsuits against the state.

A number of independent advocacy groups grew from these early experiences and they saw themselves as being engaged in a war with the health care system. Their activities included publishing polemics against psychiatric institutions and organizing 'jailbreaks' of patients held against their will.

The Netherlands, Sweden and Denmark were among the first countries in Europe to gain independent advocacy movements. In the 1970s many psychiatric hospitals in the Netherlands appointed ombudsmen to deal with patient complaints and, by the 1980s, the Board of the National Foundation for Patients' Advocates had been established. This board was funded to employ independent advocates who were appointed to all psychiatric hospitals. Similarly, Sweden had patient ombudsmen employed exclusively for handling patients' complaints. Spain also has developed a movement devoted to the well-being of patients, the Servicio de Atencion al Paciente en el Hospital, although it is not self-consciously an advocacy (defensa del paciente) movement (Hernando, 1989).

The UK advocacy movement developed under the influence of the Dutch and American experience (Gostin joined the UK mental health organization MIND in the early 1970s). In 1971, MIND launched a campaign whose aims included the development of an independent advocacy system, and in 1982 Advocacy Alliance was formed. This was an alliance of voluntary groups working with people with mental health problems and learning disabilities (Sang and O'Brien, 1984). From these developments, a well-organized independent advocacy system has grown in the fields of mental health and learning disability.

There has also been a growth of advocacy organisations at the European level. In 1991 a European Network of Users and ex-Users (of Mental Health Systems) was set up and held its first meeting in the Netherlands. It has met since at various European sites. Its main aims are to fight against discrimination and psychiatric malpractice, as well as for decent housing, work opportunities and so forth (Van der Male, 1995). It appears that the drive for advocacy has been strongest in Northern Europe.

Nursing advocacy

The idea of nurses as patients' advocates has emerged in the last 20 years and, again, the main impetus was from the USA (Mallick, 1997, p. 131). In 1973 the International Council of Nurses included advocacy in their ethical code (ICN, 1973). Interestingly, this was the first year that the same code dropped its requirement of obedience to doctors (Snowball, 1996, p. 68). Similarly, the 1976 American Nurses' Associations *Code for Nurses* omitted statements requiring obedience and adopted the idea of advocacy (Bernal, 1992, p. 18).

In the UK advocacy has become increasingly prevalent in the literature, having first appeared around fifteen years ago. The former statutory body for nursing in the UK, the UKCC, also formalized advocacy. Although the term did not appear in its code (UKCC, 1992), it did appear in the interpretative document associated with the code (UKCC, 1989). This states that there is a clear expectation 'that the practitioner will accept a role as advocate on behalf of his or her patient/clients' (p. 12).

The new statutory body, the Nursing and Midwifery Council (NMC), seems not yet to have developed a position on advocacy. Its website (www.nmc-uk.org), accessed in August 2002, uses the earlier UKCC document and refers to the previous rather than the most recent code of professional conduct (NMC, 2002). However, there seems no reason to expect its position on advocacy to be different from that of the UKCC. In the absence of any new position from the NMC, therefore, I shall assume it has the same attitude as the previous body; hence, I shall refer to the UKCC documents on advocacy in this chapter.

The idea of nursing advocacy appears to be stronger in the UK than in other areas of Europe. However, it has had some influence in countries such as Sweden and Norway (Segesten, 1993; Segesten and Fagring, 1996). In these Northern European countries there seems to be a shared vision of nurses and doctors in some form of disharmony, with nurses adopting the role of 'protecting' the patient from the inappropriate or clumsy interventions of doctors (Udén *et al.*, 1992). Such a view does not seem to be shared in Southern Europe. Spain has literature relating to the protection of patients' rights, but the emphasis is on all professionals having a duty to know and to respect patients' rights (Sànchez, 1992). An interesting book from Greece is noteworthy in that while it documents many examples of what it terms nursing 'heroism', the examples concern 'self-sacrifice and facing up to awful situations and illnesses, rather than facing up to bad tempered and incompetent consultants' (Lanara, 1991). Thus this book presents an image of nursing that is unfashionable; advocacy does not appear as a term once.

Yet where the idea of nursing advocacy has taken root there is a tension. On the one hand advocacy has been formally acknowledged as a nursing role and welcomed by many nurses, who see it as important and one they can and do strive to fulfil (Ramcharan, 1998, p. 76). On the other hand there has been a conflicting tendency in some to deny that nurses either can or should be advocates. Some of those critics have come from the independent advocacy movement and some from within nursing. This presents an important problem. Bodies such as the UKCC (and possibly the NMC) and ICN imply that a nurse who does not act as an advocate is in breach of the respective professional codes. The critics imply that a nurse cannot or should not act in the role, or should not always do so (Willard, 1996).

The source of the problem

In this section I shall suggest that the main source of the problem lies in the different meanings given to advocacy. All agree that it is some form of pleading a cause for someone. But who is pleading what cause, and for whom?

For whom?

One difference between the independent and nursing advocacy movements is that the former began with a focus almost exclusively on those with mental health problems or learning disability, while the latter focused from the beginning on all classes of patients. However, both movements appear to share a picture of the 'advocatee' as someone with some degree of vulnerability. The thought is that such people have a cause that, without advocacy, would suffer (see 'What cause?', below).

By whom?

Gates (1994, pp. 3–7) suggests at least five types of person who may undertake advocacy. These are:

- Legal – a person with legal training undertakes this form of advocacy. They will be concerned with patients' (legal) rights, hence the type of advocacy they undertake will be what I shall term (legal) rights advocacy.
- Self – someone who advocates for herself. Sometimes groups of vulnerable people will work together to gain individual confidence for self-advocacy (Simons, 1992, p. 5).
- Class – an organization advocates for a group of people with some shared status (e.g. Age Concern).

- Citizen – an individual citizen advocates for another individual. Sometimes the connection between the two individuals is made by the organizations involved in class advocacy.
- Nurse – a nurse advocates for a patient.

Other writers offer variations on this theme and the list itself is not exhaustive. For example, social workers, doctors and even pharmacists have claimed the role (Jecker, 1990; Schulz, 1991; Orentlicher, 1995; Neuberger, 1998). There is clearly some potential conflict here. Furthermore, independent advocates are often critical of the idea that professionals can perform the function.

What cause?

All advocates share the idea of pleading a cause, but the definitions of 'cause' vary. While some focus on the idea of one person representing the interests of another, as if it were his own interest (Gostin in Sang and O'Brien, 1984, p. 5), others focus on defending patients' rights (Gates, 1994, p. 2), or on assisting the patient to find meaning and purpose in life (Gadow, 1980, pp. 85ff.) and so on. These various definitions seem to fit three broad types: rights, beneficence and autonomy advocacy.

Rights advocacy

With rights advocacy the 'cause' is the patient's rights. A rights advocate ensures that a patient receives his full quota of rights, for example, by ensuring the patient and others involved in his or her care are aware of those rights, and by protecting them against threatened violation. For instance, a rights advocate would make sure a patient was aware that he or she could refuse treatment, that they were properly informed about treatment and, if they did refuse, that such a refusal was respected.

Beneficence advocacy

With beneficence advocacy, the 'cause' is the good of the patient, usually described in terms of what is in the patient's 'interest'; thus a beneficence advocate ensures that those of her acts and omissions that affect a patient are in the patient's interest. For example, a beneficence advocate might argue that it is wrong to attempt to resuscitate someone who is old, frail and dying.

Autonomy advocacy

With autonomy advocacy the 'cause' is the patient's autonomy. An autonomy advocate ensures that her acts and omissions are either the means to, or constitutive of, the patient's autonomy. For example, as means to the patient's autonomy, she or he would give a patient adequate information in order to make decisions; as constitutive of the patient's autonomy, he or she would support the patient in the decisions made.

Do all definitions of advocacy fall under these three types?

Is there an important definition of advocacy that does not fall into one of the three types, or in other words, some other 'cause' that an advocate might plead? To answer this, it is useful to compare this typology with an alternative. Falk and Adeline (1995, pp. 26ff.) suggest five types of advocacy. These are:

1. Simplistic advocacy: where one pleads the cause of another or 'does things for patients'. This notion seems underspecified and it is unclear exactly what a simplistic advocate would do for a patient. However, the notion of doing things for patients probably implies beneficence advocacy.
2. Paternalistic advocacy: where one seeks to do good for patients without seeking their consent. Falk and Adeline recognize this as being based on beneficence; hence it fits beneficence advocacy comfortably.
3. Consumer advocacy: where the advocate provides the patient with the information needed to make a decision and then withdraws (so as not to bias the decision). Falk and Adeline relate this to the patient's right to information, services and participation in decision-making. This, then, seems to be rights advocacy.

4. Consumer-centric advocacy: this is consumer advocacy plus support. In other words, the advocate will ensure that the patient gets his rights to information, services and participation in decision-making and will then support the decision the patient makes. This seems to combine rights with autonomy advocacy. A similar combination is seen in definitions that see the nurse advocate acting as a 'go-between' in respect of patients and doctors, translating medical jargon for the former and making sure the latter is aware of the patients' desires (Burnard and Chapman, 1993, p. 18).

5. Existential and human advocacy: this is advocacy as the 'philosophical foundation' of nursing and derives from the work of Gadow (1980) and Curtin (1979). Gadow is careful to demarcate existential advocacy from paternalism (beneficence advocacy) and rights advocacy. She states that existential advocacy

> is the effort to help persons *become clear about what they want* to do, by helping them discern and clarify their values in the situation, and, on the basis of that self-examination, to reach decisions which express their reaffirmed, perhaps recreated, complex of values. (Gadow, 1980, p. 85)

Whilst this looks like autonomy advocacy, it seems different from the usual autonomy-style definitions that stress only pleading what the patient wants. The key difference is in the role of clarifying values. An existential advocate does not simply seek to ensure that patients get what they want; but also ensures that what the patients want is authentic. This is still a form of autonomy advocacy, but the difference from the more common type of autonomy advocacy lies in ambiguities within the notion of autonomy itself. These ambiguities will be examined below under the heading of 'Autonomy advocacy'.

Thus, in the absence of any counter-examples, I shall assume that the suggestion that all definitions of advocacy can be categorized into at least one of the three types suggested is plausible.

In the next sections I shall suggest that the main source of the conflicts concerning advocacy lie in the different notions of 'cause' that the advocate pleads, and two main problems can be identified. The first is that none of the types is unambiguous. This means that, for example, it would not be clear what a nurse claiming to uphold a patient's autonomy, or rights, would be doing. The second is that the three types of advocacy are different and have the potential to conflict.

This means that, for example, a nurse acting as advocate for a patient's autonomy and interest may have to plead two opposing causes. I shall examine these two problems in turn.

Problem 1: Internal ambiguities in the three types of advocacy

Rights advocacy (Bandman and Bandman, 1995, p. 18)

The rights advocate ensures that the patient receives his full quota of rights; but what are those rights? In the first place we know that a right is some form of entitlement. We also know that it is related to duty. Thus negative rights imply a duty to leave someone alone, whereas positive rights imply a duty to provide someone with a service. Lastly we know that rights are indefeasible; that is, they cannot be overridden for reasons of, say, another person's utility. Hence you have the right not to be killed even if many hundreds of people would benefit from your death.

However, there is an important distinction between legal and moral rights (Gillon, 1992, pp. 55–56). Legal rights are enforceable: if someone fails to perform a positive or negative duty in relation to your legal rights, then you have recourse to the civil or criminal courts. Relevant examples in health care include the right not to be killed and the right not to be treated without consent. Moral rights are far more slippery. The idea is that everyone has certain 'human rights' such as the right not to be killed or the right to free speech. One problem with this notion is that it is tempting to describe anything good as a moral right. Hence we are told that people have a moral right to clean water, a decent job or a house.

Moral rights are not necessarily legal rights. For example, the right to free speech is not a legal right in China, the right to shelter is not a legal right in the UK, yet both may be considered by some to be moral rights. With what type of right, then, is rights advocacy concerned? The answer seems to be with both. For example, legal advocacy will be concerned solely with someone's legal rights. But class advocates may well campaign to get what they regard as moral rights enshrined in law.

Can nurses be rights advocates?

This question is ambiguous between 'Are nurses able to perform rights advocacy?' and 'Are nurses likely to be successful in achieving the outcome of rights advocacy?' I shall assume that a positive answer to both these questions is necessary in order to affirm that nurses can be rights advocates.

Where nurses describe themselves as undertaking rights advocacy they seem to be thinking mainly of legal rights, in particular, issues surrounding consent. This is probably to the good for two reasons. The first is that legal rights are fairly unambiguous and hence the goal of legal rights advocacy is clear. The second is that nurses are reasonably well placed to undertake this form of advocacy within a limited framework. Nurses are able to respect patients' legal rights themselves and are able to raise objections should others threaten to violate those legal rights.

On first appearance it looks as though what this amounts to is that nurses will not break the law and will try to stop others from doing so. While this may sound fairly trivial, it is a serious role. Unfortunately patients can suffer violations of their legal rights and nurses have successfully undertaken the role of legal rights advocates where such abuse occurs or is threatened (for example by ensuring consent is properly informed).

Undertaking *moral* rights advocacy is more problematic. In the first place it is unclear what moral rights are; if they are not already enshrined in law then it is likely that their status as moral rights will be disputed (such as the right to housing). As well as this, it is unclear how a nurse could help someone exercise moral rights that are not recognized legally. For instance, how would a nurse ensure that a homeless person is given a home? However, through their professional organizations (see Arndt's chapter, Chapter 5 in this volume), nurses can act as lobbyists to try and get moral rights enshrined in law.

Do nurses have a special claim to be rights advocates?

By 'special claim' it is intended that nurses are able to perform this role better than, or to the exclusion of, others in the health care team. As far as legal rights advocacy is concerned, the law would expect all health care professionals to respect patients' legal rights. Nurses, like all health care professionals, should be legal rights advocates.

Given that nurses are not well placed to be moral rights advocates, it follows that they have no special claim to the role. As 'lobbyists' for moral rights they are, at most, as well placed as other health care professionals.

Beneficence advocacy

The beneficence advocate ensures that any acts and omissions that affect a patient are in the patient's interest. Here, it is the term 'interest' that creates a problem. Dworkin (1993, pp. 201ff.) points to two ways in which the concept of 'interest' is used.

1. Experiential interest – it is in someone's experiential interest to have pleasant experiences and avoid painful ones. Someone acting as an advocate of experiential interest might, for example, ensure that a child gets adequate post-operative pain control.
2. Critical interest – it is in someone's critical interest to live, and have lived, a good life. For a hedonist there is no difference between experiential and critical interest: a good life is simply one with maximum pleasure and minimum pain. But for most of us a good life is more than the sum of pleasant over painful experiences. For example, if we say that it harms someone's interests to be kept alive in a persistent vegetative state, or to be cuckolded without ever realizing, then we acknowledge the existence of critical interests.

It is critical interests that create most problems for beneficence advocacy. Deciding what is in someone's critical interest requires a coherent view about what constitutes a good life. Such decisions are most commonly formulated in terms of quality-of-life judgements. It is important not to confuse beneficence with autonomy advocacy in such cases. Take the example of a patient in persistent vegetative state and the question of whether he or she should be kept alive by artificial feeding. One way we could decide would be by 'substituted judgement' whereby we would seek to find out what the patient would have wanted. Another way would be by 'interests'; we would seek to do what we thought best for the patient. The former method appeals to the principle of respecting autonomy, the latter to beneficence.

Beneficence advocacy employs the latter method: it pleads the cause of the patient in terms of what is thought good for her, not necessarily what she wants or would have wanted.

Can nurses be beneficence advocates?

Beneficence advocacy appears to be commonly reported by nurses when describing acts of advocacy (Teasdale in 'Nursing Forum', 1996, p. 656). The clearest cases where nurses have thought themselves to be acting as beneficence advocates concern incompetent patients, such as babies, the unconscious, or the severely senile. These cases involve both experiential interest and critical interest. For example, neonatal nurses have been influential in pleading for greater analgesia in neonatology (experiential interest) and in pleading that treatment be withdrawn for neonates facing an appalling quality of life (critical interest) (cf. Spence, 1998). Thus nurses can and do undertake beneficence advocacy of both types.

Do nurses have a special claim to be beneficence advocates?

For both beneficence and autonomy advocacy the argument is occasionally put that nurses gain privileged knowledge of the patient, which enables them to see either what is good for the patient (beneficence) or what the patient wants (autonomy). A number of counterpoints could be made. First, it might be claimed that the doctor's additional knowledge means that he or she may have a better handle on what is good for the patient. Second, what is the source of the nurse's supposed superior knowledge? It is sometimes said it is her 24-hour contact with the patient, but no nurse has such contact with a patient. Given understaffed wards and shift patterns of working, the time a nurse spends with each individual patient can be fairly short. In addition, the sort of casual banter that goes on between patient and nurse over a bed-bath hardly entitles the latter to claim intimate knowledge of the patient (because quality of contact time matters more than quantity). Third, there is little evidence of this supposed privileged knowledge. Thus there seems no obvious reason why nurses are able to plead the cause of the patient's interest better than any other health care professional.

Autonomy advocacy (Rumbold, 1993, p. 211; Simons, 1993, p. 14)

The autonomy advocate ensures that her acts and omissions respect patients' autonomy. Unfortunately the term 'autonomy' is also ambiguous (cf. Yeo, cited in Mallick, 1997, p. 133). One can discern two broad approaches: one focusing on acts, the other on agents.

1. Act-focused approaches define autonomy in terms of the criteria necessary to deem an act autonomous. Autonomy is seen as a quality that belongs to an act when certain criteria are fulfilled. For example, an act may be deemed autonomous if it is performed intentionally, with a certain level of understanding, and in the absence of controlling influences (Beauchamp and Faden, 1986, p. 238). On such accounts, an autonomy advocate would plead that autonomous acts are respected. For instance, she would plead that a patient be allowed to return home if that was what he or she desired. An autonomy advocate would also try to help facilitate such acts by, for example, arranging transport and occupational therapy.
2. Agent-focused approaches define autonomy in terms of the criteria necessary to deem an agent autonomous. Autonomy is a quality belonging to such agents. For example, an agent might be called autonomous where he or she has the ability to form second-order preferences by reflecting on first-order preferences (Dworkin, 1988, p. 15) or where able to make rational decisions that reflect personal values and character (an Aristotelian account). It is less clear what respect for autonomy involves in these accounts, but roughly it is that one should facilitate and/or not interfere with the acts of autonomous agents.

A key difference between the two is that act approaches tend to be less demanding. Take the case of an 18-year-old man who has taken an overdose after being rejected by his lover. He refuses life-saving treatment because he cannot see the point of living without her.

An act-centred approach might deem his act autonomous and thus worthy of respect: it is intentional, performed with sufficient knowledge (he knows he will die without treatment), and is without controlling influences (no one is forcing him to refuse treatment). An autonomy advocate acting with this model of autonomy would have to plead that the benighted teenager is not treated. Certainly in UK law it would appear that the teenager is sufficiently autonomous, hence his wish should be respected (Kennedy and Grubb, 1994, ch. 3). As such, a 'legal rights' advocate would also be committed to pleading the non-treatment cause.

An agent-centred approach may be more doubtful. Dworkin's account would question whether this man is properly able to reflect on first-order preferences at this time. An Aristotelian account would question whether his action reflects his values and character. An autonomy advocate on this account would be more likely to try to get the agent to 'see reason' rather than plead that he is not treated.

We can now see why both Gadow's account of existential advocacy and the more basic accounts centred on supporting patients' decisions can be described as autonomy types even though they seem very different. It is because the former adopts an agent-centred approach to advocacy, while the latter adopts an act-centred approach.

Can nurses be autonomy advocates?

Many criticisms of the notion of nurse advocacy are aimed at autonomy advocacy. There seem to be a number of situations in which it would not be possible. For example, a nurse would be unable to plead the alcoholic's autonomous desire for another drink (Allmark and Klarzynski, 1992, p. 34; cf. Kendrick, 1994, 1998). However, it might be argued that this is an act-centred approach to autonomy and that the nurse could act as an advocate on an agent-centred approach. Thus, for example, the alcoholic could be compared with the 18-year-old overdose patient who is asking for something which is not arising from his true, autonomous self. This would be hard to maintain. The 18-year-old is suffering from a temporary aberration, is acting 'out of character'. The alcoholic's desire for a drink is 'in character' and is autonomous from both the act and agent viewpoints.

It seems, then, that nurses cannot consistently be autonomy advocates. In most cases we are required by law to respect people's autonomy anyway; for example, we are usually unable to treat without consent. But in cases where the law allows or insists that we do not respect people's autonomy, such as when holding psychiatric patients against their will, or preventing confused patients from leaving a ward, the nurse will be unable to plead the autonomy cause on either act or agent accounts of autonomy. It follows from this that nurses do not have any special claim to be autonomy advocates.

In summary, then, even if nurses were clear about in which of the three types of advocacy they were employed, there would be problems. Do we plead for moral or legal rights and, if the former, what are they? Do we plead for critical or experiential interests and, if so, what are they? Do we plead for respecting patient's act- or agent-centred autonomy? None the less, it seems clear that nurses should at least act as legal rights advocates and benefience advocates. It is less obvious that they should act as moral rights advocates.

Acting as autonomy advocates presents far greater problems. First, one must decide to what notion of autonomy one is appealing. I have suggested that act and agent notions of autonomy will suggest different 'causes' for the nurse to plead. Second, whatever notion the nurse employs, there will be times when the nurse is unable to plead the cause as autonomy advocacy will conflict with other nursing roles.

Problem 2: Conflicts between the three types of advocacy

In this section I wish to defend the following argument:

1. Many definitions of advocacy fall into *more than one* of the three types.
2. The term 'interests' has further ambiguities that allow many apparently beneficence-type definitions of advocacy to be interpreted also as either autonomy or rights types.
3. The UKCC's definition of advocacy is a beneficence type that is open to precisely this type of dual interpretation. This is of particular importance if I am correct in assuming that the NMC shares the same beliefs about advocacy as the UKCC.
4. The three definitions are distinct and would, in some situations, be in opposition.
5. Thus in some situations it is not possible for someone to be simultaneously an autonomy, beneficence, and rights advocate.
6. Therefore definitions that fall into more than one type are invalid, while those that are open to dual interpretation (such as the UKCC's) are invalid unless properly clarified. By 'invalid' it is meant

that a practitioner would be unable to be an advocate of such a category.

This argument consists of four premises (1–4) and two conclusions (5–6). I believe the argument is logically sound, although it requires one or two uncontroversial premises in addition to those already stated. As such, if the premises are true, then the conclusions are true also. Let us, now, examine the premises.

1   Many definitions fall into more than one of the three types

I have already suggested that 'consumer-centric' advocacy combines rights with autonomy advocacy (e.g. Brower, cited in Cahill, 1994, p. 371). There are also definitions that conflate rights with beneficence advocacy (Sang and O'Brien, 1984, p. 9; Thompson *et al.*, 1994, pp. 94–95) and definitions that conflate beneficence and autonomy advocacy (Murphy and Hunter, cited in Kendrick, 1998, p. 227). There is at least one definition that conflates all three. This is due to Clark (1988), who states that advocacy is

> informing the patient of his rights in a particular situation, making sure he has all the necessary information to make an informed decision, supporting him in the decision he makes, and protecting and safeguarding his interests. (Cited in Sawyer, 1988, p. 28)

2   The term 'interests' has further ambiguities

Many definitions of advocacy focus on the interests of the patient. I have already pointed to the problem of whether we intend experiential or critical interests when we use the term, but there are at least two further ambiguities of note.

The first is that people's rights are sometimes identified with their interests. For example, 'nurses have a responsibility to protect the rights of those patients who are unable for whatever reason to look after their own interests' (Wells, cited in Cahill, 1994, p. 371). Thus a nurse may think that having regard for someone's interest is simply having regard for their rights and, hence, interpret a beneficence definition of advocacy as a rights one and *vice versa*. This is an error. We do not have a right to whatever is in our interest; for example, we do not have the right to housing (legally at least). Neither are all rights necessarily in our interest, such as the right not to be killed, as this is a right that we cannot surrender even if it were to be in our interest to be killed by, say, euthanasia.

The second ambiguity is that people's interests are sometimes identified with what they want, and thus with their autonomy as noted by Willard (1996, p. 62). In this sense, the alcoholic has an interest in obtaining another drink, and were we to identify interests with desires in this way then pleading a patient's interest would be identical to pleading their autonomous cause (on the 'act-centred' accounts of autonomy, at least). This would not be an error, but it is an important ambiguity. An alcoholic's desire for a drink may be his strongest desire, hence in this sense, his most important interest. We might, however, be reluctant to say it is 'in his interest'. What this means is that it is possible for a definition that looks unambiguously of the beneficence type to be interpreted as either a rights or autonomy type. This leads us to premise 3.

3   The UKCC's definition is open to dual interpretation

In *Exercising Accountability* (UKCC, 1989) the UKCC seems to embrace beneficence advocacy. It says that although the *Code of Professional Conduct* (UKCC, 1992) does not explicitly state the role of advocate, it is implicit in the introductory paragraphs and 'several of its clauses'. It then defines advocacy as being 'concerned with promoting and safeguarding the well-being and interests of patients and clients' (UKCC, 1989, p. 12). The belief that this is intended to mean beneficence advocacy is based on the conjunction of 'well-being' with 'interests', and this notion is further developed in the subsequent discussion where it is suggested that such advocacy might mean going against the wishes of relatives and parents in the case of incompetent patients. However, it is not entirely clear as some of the discussion also hints at an autonomy interpretation.

The lack of clarity is more manifest in the document that updates *Exercising Accountability*, *Guidelines for Professional Practice* (UKCC, 1996). In the latter, the section that deals with advocacy is entitled 'Patient and client advocacy and autonomy' (p. 13). The link between the two concepts is not made explicit, for instance, by saying that advocacy involves supporting and fostering patients' autonomy, but it is implicit in at least three ways. First, it tells us that the practitioner must not practise 'in a way which assumes that only they know what is best for the patient or client...'. Second, the discussion refers to clause 5 of the *Code of Professional Conduct*, which is concerned with fostering autonomy. Third, the definition of advocacy drops the reference to 'well-being' and goes on to say that 'Advocacy also involves providing support if the patient refuses treatment/care or withdraws their consent' (p. 13). If only the 1996 document were in existence, then it would seem fairly clear that the UKCC intended an autonomy definition of advocacy. As it is, the presence of the term 'interests' in the 1996 definition, and the existence of the 1989 document, raise the suspicion that both beneficence and autonomy advocacy are intended.

4 The three types are distinct and may be opposed

Consider the following case and ask, what would the nurse advocate do?

> A 52-year-old man with motor neurone disease is admitted to intensive care after a suicide attempt, but refuses all life-support. He is alert and expresses to the house officers his strong belief in a patient's right to die with dignity. He says that his progressive physical disabilities are making his life unbearable and asks that his life be ended. Told this is not possible, he insists that he does not want vigorous medical intervention should serious complications develop.

As a legal rights advocate the nurse will, having ensured that the man is competent, make certain that his desire to avoid vigorous medical intervention is respected. As a moral rights advocate the nurse may feel that there is a moral right to die and that this should include euthanasia. Pushed to the extreme, perhaps the nurse will perform the act for the patient; after all, we are told that advocacy may involve risks to health, job and elements of one's life (Williams, cited in Duxbury, 1996, p. 38).

As beneficence advocate the nurse will want to plead the patient's interest. His experiential interest is unclear: perhaps there are pleasures ahead that the man has not predicted, or the pains are over-estimated. The nurse would need to weigh the probable pleasures and pains before deciding what to advocate. His critical interest appears to be in being killed, or at least being allowed to die, but the 'critical interests advocate' may have some doubts. The nurse may think that the man has made the wrong assessment of quality of life and thus not support his choice but instead try to persuade him against it.

If the nurse is acting as autonomy advocate, the case depends on the notion of autonomy the nurse is using. On an act-centred account the man's choices seem clearly autonomous. But on a richer agent-centred account of autonomy the advocate may have some doubts, for although his choice may be voluntary, one must ask if it truly reflects the man.

In this case, then, the nurse as advocate may be pulled in many different directions. As rights and as act-centred autonomy advocate she might plead not to treat aggressively or to actively kill the patient, while as agent-centred autonomy or as beneficence advocate, the nurse might oppose the man's own choice.

I have defended the four premises of the argument set out at the beginning of this section. If I am right, then the two conclusions follow. In some situations nurses cannot simultaneously be an autonomy, beneficence and rights advocate, and definitions that suggest they can are invalid.

Conclusion: resolving the problem

We began with a problem: in many countries, nurses are frequently told that they can and must be patient advocates, but they are also told this is impossible or undesirable. The source of this problem lies in the multiple possible interpretations of the 'cause' that the advocate is supposed to plead. The nurse can and should act as a legal rights advocate: not to do so would violate both the law and their professional codes. The nurse should also act as the advocate for a patient's interest, although this needs to be tempered by respect for the patient's autonomy (as required by law) and by concern for other patients. It is not possible for the nurse to act as advocate for the patient's autonomy (either act or agent). Usually nurses will respect patients' autonomy when they respect their legal rights. But whenever a patient's autonomy is not supported by law, then nurses are likely to find it very problematic to plead their cause, such as in the case of a detained psychiatric patient who demands to leave.

It seems clear that those who support nurse advocacy have in mind the types of advocacy the nurse can fulfil, particularly legal rights advocacy. Those who oppose nurse advocacy have in mind the types that nurses cannot fulfil, particularly autonomy advocacy. Having identified the source of the problem, can we resolve it?

One way to resolve the argument would be to identify the correct definition of advocacy and ask whether nurses can perform it. Thus, if we said that advocacy was 'legal rights' advocacy, we could say that nurses both can and should perform it, and that they are reasonably well placed to do so. Alternatively, if autonomy advocacy is 'right', then nurses cannot perform it. This is the position I once took (Allmark and Klarzynski, 1992). I no longer think this is correct. Historically the term advocacy has been associated primarily with legal rights advocacy as practised by lawyers. However, it is clear that the term has developed beyond that in the ways I have described. Furthermore, that development has not just been down to nurses. The independent advocacy movement is also fond of autonomy, beneficence and moral rights advocacy (Sang and O'Brien, 1984 *passim,* Simons, 1993, p. 14). As such it would be wrong and impractical to try to reimpose one specific meaning on the term.

A second resolution would involve saying that the term 'advocacy' is ambiguous and unhelpful. Nurses need to know they must support patients' legal rights and what this involves, such as usually respecting patients' choices. They should know that it is important always to act with the patient's interest in mind (within the limits of both the law and available resources). But naming these things 'advocacy' adds little. Furthermore, its use can and does cause confusion and conflict. Therefore, we should remove advocacy from our discussions.

A third resolution would be to say that 'advocacy' is ambiguous, but helpful. The problems we have in defining advocacy and related terms such as autonomy, and the problems we have in *being* advocates, are moral problems, the problems of doing right by our patients and clients. Furthermore, taking on the mantle of advocacy acts as a constant reminder to us of the sort of priorities we have in practice. I have yet to hear a nurse tell me of an act of 'advocacy' that I thought was wrong, even if I thought it was incorrectly described as advocacy.

There may be other resolutions. My own favoured one would be the second: for nursing and other health care professions to drop the use of the term and to focus instead on a different model of ethical conduct.

Acknowledgements

I have benefited from the perceptive comments of Paul Ramcharan on an earlier draft. Thanks also to Win Tadd, Professor Da Silva, Professor Lorensen and Diana Frederiksen.

References

Allmark, P. and Klarzynski, R. (1992) 'The case against nurse advocacy', *British Journal of Nursing*, **2**: 33–36.

Bandman, E. and Bandman, B. (1995) *Nursing Ethics Through the Life Span*, 3rd edn, London: Prentice-Hall.

Beauchamp, T. and Faden, R. (1986) *A History and Theory of Informed Consent*, New York: Oxford University Press.

Bernal, E. (1992) 'The nurse as patient advocate', *Hastings Center Report*, **22** (4): 18–23.

Brendon, D. (1991) *Innovation Without Change*, London: Macmillan.

Brower, H. (1982) 'Advocacy: what is it?', *Journal of Gerontological Nursing*, **8**: 141–143.

Burnard, P. and Chapman, C. (1993) *Professional and Ethical Issues in Nursing*, 2nd edn, London: Scutari.

Cahill, J. (1994) 'Are you prepared to be their advocate?', *Professional Nurse*, **9**: 371–375.

Curtin, L. (1979) 'The nurse as advocate: a philosophical foundation for nursing', *Advances in Nursing Science*, **1**: 1–10.

Duxbury, J. (1996) 'The nurse's role as patient advocate for mentally ill people', *Nursing Standard*, **10** (20): 36–39.

Dworkin, G. (1988) *The Theory and Practice of Autonomy*, Cambridge: Cambridge University Press.

Dworkin, R. (1993) *Life's Dominion*, London: HarperCollins.

Falk, R. and Adeline, R. (1995) 'Advocacy and empowerment: dichotomous or synchronous concepts?', *Advances in Nursing Science*, **18**(2): 25–32.

Gadow, S. (1980) 'Existential advocacy: philosophical foundation of nursing', in Spicker, S. and Gadow, S. (eds) *Nursing Images and Ideals*, New York: Springer, pp. 79–101.

Gates, B. (1994) *Advocacy: A Nurses' Guide*, London: Scutari.

Gillon, R. (1992) *Philosophical Medical Ethics*, 2nd edn, Chichester: Wiley.

Hernando, P. (1989) 'Servicio de Atencion al Paciente en el Hospital', *Todo Hospital*, **62**: 67–70.

ICN (1973) *Code for Nurses: Ethical Concepts Applied to Nursing*, Geneva: ICN.

Jecker, N. (1990) 'Integrating medical ethics with normative theory: patient advocacy and social responsibility', *Theoretical Medicine*, **11**: 125–129.

Kendrick, K. (1994) 'An advocate for whom – doctor or patient?', *Professional Nurse*, **9**: 826–829.

Kendrick, K. (1998) 'Ethical issues in critical care nursing', in Tadd, W. (ed.) *Ethical Issues in Nursing and Midwifery Practice – Perspectives from Europe*, London: Macmillan, pp. 171–232.

Kennedy, I. and Grubb, A. (1994) *Medical Law – text with materials*, 2nd edn, London: Butterworths.

Lanara, V. (1991) *Heroism as a Nursing Value*, Athens: University of Athens.

Mallick, M. (1997) 'Advocacy in nursing – a review of the literature', *Journal of Advanced Nursing*, **25**: 130–138.

Neuberger, J. (1998) 'Patients' priorities', *British Medical Journal*, **317**: 260–262.

NMC (Nursing and Midwifery Council) (2002) *Code of Professional Conduct*, London: NMC.

'Nursing Forum' (1996) 'Can a nurse be a patient's advocate?', *Professional Nurse*, **11**: 655–658.

Orentlicher, D. (1995) 'Physician advocacy for patients under managed care', *Journal of Clinical Ethics*, **6**: 333–334.

Ramcharan, P. (1998) *Fostering a Culture of Civil Rights*, Report to Gwynedd Community Trust, Learning Disability Service.

Rumbold, G. (1993) *Ethics in nursing practice*, 2nd edn, London: Baillière Tindall.

Sànchez, J. (1992) 'La Profesionalización en los Servicios de Atención al Usuario', in proceedings of *VI Congreso de la Sociedad Espanôla de Atención al Usuario de la Sanidad*, pp. 4–5.

Sang, B. and O'Brien, J. (1984) 'Advocacy – the UK and American Experiences', *King's Fund Project Paper no. 51*, London: King Edward's Hospital Fund for London.

Sawyer, J. (1988) 'On behalf of the patient', *Nursing Times*, **84** (41): 28–29.

Schulz, R. (1991) 'The pharmacists role in patient care', *Hastings Center Report*, **21** (1): 12–17.

Segesten, K. (1993) 'Patient advocacy – an important part of the daily work of the expert nurse', *Scholarly Inquiry for Nursing Practice*, **7**: 129–135.

Segesten, K. and Fagring, A. (1996) 'Patient advocacy – an essential part of quality nursing care', *International Nursing Review*, **43** (5): 142–144.

Simons, K. (1992) *Sticking up for yourself*, York: Rowntree.

Simons, K. (1993) *Citizen Advocacy: the Inside View*, Bristol: Norah Fry Research Centre/University of Bristol.

Snowball, J. (1996) 'Asking nurses about advocating for patients: "reactive" and "proactive" accounts', *Journal of Advanced Nursing*, **24**: 67–75.

Spence, K. (1998) 'Ethical issues for neonatal nurses', *Nursing Ethics*, **5**: 206–217.

Thompson, I., Melia, K. and Boyd, K. (1994) *Nursing Ethics*, Edinburgh: Churchill Livingstone.

Udén, G., Norberg, A., Lindseth, A. and Marhaug, V. (1992) 'Ethical reasoning in nurses' and physicians' stories about care episodes', *Journal of Advanced Nursing*, **17**: 1028–1034.

UKCC (1989) *Exercising Accountability*, London: UKCC.

UKCC (1992) *Code of Professional Conduct*, London: UKCC.

UKCC (1996) *Guidelines for Professional Practice*, London: UKCC.

Van der Male, R. (1995) 'Client movement in Europe', *Seishin Shinkeigaku Zasshi*, **97** (7): 517–521.

Willard, C. (1996) 'The nurse's role as patient advocate: obligation or imposition?', *Journal of Advanced Nursing*, **24**: 60–66.

9

How Effective are Codes of Nursing Ethics?

Andrew Edgar

Introduction

Any enquiry into the effectiveness of professional codes of ethics requires that a number of presuppositions are made explicit. For example, effectiveness can only be assessed in terms of a clear account of the objectives that the code is expected to fulfil. More profoundly, precisely because any code is a written text – and thus a document that must make sense to practitioners, to their employers and managers, and to their clients and the general public – there are what may be called 'hermeneutic' conditions that the text must meet.[1] This means that codes must be so written as to be capable of precise (although not necessarily uncontestable or uncontroversial) interpretation.

Summary

The purpose of this chapter is to explore the problems that are encountered in any attempt, on the one hand, to establish clearly the objectives that codes may be expected to fulfil, and on the other, to establish precise interpretations of codes. It will be argued that many nursing codes are ineffective in achieving any intended objective, precisely because they fail to satisfy certain conditions of readability. It will be argued also that confusions over the objectives and the contexts within which codes are intended to be read lead to ambiguities, so that codes fail to provide a framework within which practitioners (or indeed any

155

other reader) could challenge, explore and ultimately make sense of their own moral conduct.[2]

Interpreting the ICN code

Although the International Council of Nurses (ICN) has published a 2000 edition of its code, discussion will centre on the earlier versions, as these clearly demonstrate the changing values and professional aspirations important to the discussions in this chapter. In addition, little has changed in the 2000 edition.

The 1973 edition of the ICN *Code of Ethics* begins with the following statement: 'The fundamental responsibility of the nurse is fourfold: to promote health, to prevent illness, to restore health and to alleviate suffering' (ICN, 1973, p. 1). The statement is seemingly unambiguous. Its meaning is apparently clear, and indeed, like the rest of the code, it is written in a plain style that should serve to make interpretation unproblematic. Yet, in interpreting this, as any other statement, we must make certain presuppositions, for example, about the context within which the statement is made, and the intentions of the speaker or writer. The same words, uttered in different circumstances, can mean very different things. Alasdair MacIntyre offers the following illustration, which highlights the problem. 'I am standing waiting for a bus and the young man standing next to me suddenly says: "The name of the common wild duck is *Histrionicus histrionicus histrionicus*." There is no problem as to the meaning of the sentence he uttered: the problem is, how to understand the question, what was he doing in uttering it?' (MacIntyre, 1981, p. 195).

In reading the ICN's statement, we make a number of assumptions (perhaps unwittingly) about the context and intention of the code's authors. To begin to explicate these assumptions, one may look at the opening statement in the wider context of the code itself.[3] The statement is part of a section within the code entitled 'Ethical concepts applied to nursing'. This is already problematic, for the opening statement is not obviously moral in tone. It is, rather, a broad assertion of the general purposes that nursing serves. It is grouped with statements that have a more overt moral content. These include the problematic claim that: 'The need for nursing is universal' (ICN, 1973, p. 1). Further statements refer to the nurse's respect for moral values, the importance of non-discriminatory practice, and the relationship of the nurse to other people and groups. From this, we may come to recognize these initial statements as an attempt to present the basic purposes of nursing in a moral light. Thus, just as *'Histrionicus histrionicus histrionicus'* comes to make sense as a reply to the question, 'What is the Latin name of the common wild duck?', so we may understand the ICN statements as the answer to an implicit question. This question might be formulated along the following lines: 'What, morally, is entailed in being a nurse?'; or 'How am I to understand myself, morally, as a nurse?'

Yet, even if we have explicitly formulated this question, we have not done with the problem of interpreting the code. The fact that the ICN statement is banal cannot be avoided. Even as an answer to an enquiry about the moral character of nursing, it is little more than a statement of what now is obvious. This raises the problem of why, or more precisely, in what circumstances, the original question needed to be asked. Questions themselves only make sense in certain contexts, so, for example, enquiries about Latin names from strangers in bus queues are anything but unproblematically meaningful. A full understanding of the ICN code therefore presupposes some notion of who should ask this question and why. An answer to this problem may lie in an earlier edition of the ICN code.

In the original 1953 edition of the ICN code, the following statements can be found:

> (6) A nurse recognises not only the responsibilities but also the limitations of her or his professional functions; recommends or gives medical treatment without medical order only in emergencies and reports such action to a physician at the earliest possible moment. (7) The nurse is under an obligation to carry out the physician's orders intelligently and loyally and to refuse to participate in unethical procedures. (8) The nurse sustains confidence in the physician and other members of the health teams: incompetence or unethical conduct of associates should be exposed but only to the proper authority. (Callahan, 1988, pp. 452–453)

The 1973 edition contains the following parallel statements:

> The nurse uses judgment in relation to individual competence when accepting and delegating responsibilities. ... The nurse sustains a cooperative relationship with co-workers in the nursing and other fields. The nurse takes appropriate action to safeguard the individual when his care is endangered by a co-worker or any other person. (Davis and Aroskar, 1978, pp. 13–14)

There is nothing in the 1973 edition of the code that corresponds to the presupposed subordination of the nurse to the physician that is found in the 1953 edition. Here is the clue that may serve to highlight what is happening in these codes. The historical context within which the two editions are written has changed. The 1973 code expresses the presupposition of a greater assertiveness of the autonomy and responsibility of the nursing profession. Obedience to the physician is no longer the issue it was. Bluntly, by 1973 nursing did not need to make polite reference to the authority of the doctor. Yet the 1973 code is still making an assertion about the autonomy of nursing as a profession. The war is being won, in comparison to the cautious tone of appeasement that characterizes the 1953 position, even though victory is not yet secured. It is in the very banality of its opening statement that the strident tones of this assertion are, paradoxically, most evident. The question as to the moral self-understanding of the nurse comes from one who is sceptical about the status of nursing as a profession – or at least, the answer is addressed to such a person. A statement that is banal to the nurse is important, precisely because it may be a revelation to the sceptical and unsympathetic outsider, such as the authoritarian physician of 1953, who presupposes that the nurse is but his handmaiden.

This analysis of the interpretation of the code has answered the question of the objective of the code and has thus opened up the possibility of assessing the effectiveness of the code. On the above reading, the objective of the ICN code is not, simply, to state the moral purposes of nursing, but rather to promote the professional status of nursing in the face of overt opposition, or at best mere insensitivity, from others. In recognizing this objective, the status of the code as an ethical document may need some reassessment, albeit that this serves to clarify the ambiguous relationship of the opening statement to the ethics inherent in the other statements. Moral autonomy and the possession of a distinctive moral orientation to practise are being presented as part of what is entailed by professionalism.

This claim may be supported through the following analysis. It was suggested above that the ICN code is a response to a question along the following lines: 'What, morally, is entailed in being a nurse?' Yet, if the objective of the code is a political one, as part of the struggle for professionalization, it may be suggested that this question might be further refined thus: 'How am I to present myself, as a professional nurse, to someone who is not a nurse?' The appeal to ethics originates, on this account, not in the question, but in the reply. Indeed, the opening statement replies directly to such a question. It is only with the third statement, '[I]nherent in nursing is respect for life, dignity and rights of man', that an appeal to ethics is explicitly presented as part of a comprehensive reply. The statements grouped together as 'Ethical concepts applied to nursing' assert that the professionalism of the nurse rests, in large part, upon the possession of a moral expertise, and that this expertise surpasses that of the physician. As such, the code draws upon a traditional understanding of nursing, which runs back through the supposed example of Florence Nightingale, and at least to the tradition of Christian service to the poor and needful.[4] The ICN code further includes references to confidentiality and respect for the values of patients, and as such does much to summarize and prescribe the agenda for nursing ethics in the decades to come. Yet it also does something more subtle than this.

The account that the code provides of ethics is a distinctive one. Ethical problems and dilemmas are implicitly understood in the context of the struggle for professionalization. The ethical problems that the code highlights are primarily threats to the continuing development of professional practice. These include poor and difficult working conditions;[5] limitations in technical and other training;[6] the failings of others;[7] and the lack of professional organization and participation in that organization. The apparently excessive demands that the nurse's personal life should reflect credit upon the profession, and that nurses should fulfil their duty as citizens, may reflect the demand that the nurse should leave no hostages to fortune when professional status is still vulnerable.

Conversely, the code also invokes the personal resources that are available to combat these threats. The nurse thus 'uses judgment' in dealing with certain problems, and has a 'personal responsibility for maintaining nursing practice'. The meanings of 'judgment' and 'responsibility' are not elaborated. Yet their use may work best as an exhortation to the nurse to believe in her or his professional status and ability to maintain it.

Guidance for conduct

The ICN code is intended for an international audience, although numerous national nursing associations, especially in Europe, have taken it as their model, by broadly imitating its plain style and its structure, consisting in a preamble and a series of brief statements of principle. Thus, for example, even the lengthy American Nurses' Association (ANA, 2001) code follows this pattern, albeit with a substantial elaboration of each statement. Some codes quote passages verbatim, such as the code of the Finnish Federation of Nurses (FFN, 1997). In addition, the national codes tend to present, as the core of nursing ethics, the same issues as those found in the ICN code. These include non-discriminatory practice; confidentiality; the relationship to other health care professions, which itself can be developed into patient advocacy, as for example in the American code; the relationship between the nurse's private and professional life; the limits to the nurse's competence; and the nurse's relationship to society in general. The very similarity of national codes to the international code may be regarded as a cause of concern. Should one not expect national codes to express distinctive national problems, for instance, those arising from the organization and funding of the health care sector, as well as reflecting national values?

It has been argued above that the objective of the ICN codes was to promote the professionalization of nursing. From this it was suggested that much that is banal or trivial in the ICN codes appears so only because Western Europeans are no longer the codes' intended audience. The professional status of nursing is a fact in most, if not all, of the countries of Western Europe. This is still, of course, not the case globally. In many countries, including some in Central and Eastern Europe, the assertion still needs to be made, and to be made as part of a continuing political struggle to gain nursing the recognition and resources that it deserves. Yet, if the ICN code now has its intended audience largely outside the industrialized West, then a problem arises as to how satisfactory a model it is for the codes of developed Western countries.

This problem is compounded if it is accepted, as argued above, that the ICN code uses ethics, in the form of the distinctive moral expertise of the nurse, as part of the articulation of an account of professional nursing. The problem may be formulated, initially, along the following lines. Many national associations, implicitly or explicitly, take the objective of their codes to be the provision of a set of ethical guidelines for everyday practice. Thus the Finnish code 'is to provide support for all nurses in their everyday decision-making concerning ethical questions of nursing'. In the UK, the Royal College of Nursing claims that a code is required 'in order to make explicit those moral standards which should guide professional decisions...and in order to encourage responsible moral decision making throughout the profession'. The American code provides 'guidance for conduct and relationships in carrying out nursing responsibilities'. In itself, this objective is laudable. The problem occurs when it is recognized that the objective of the ICN codes is quite different. What the ICN codes conspicuously fail to do, on the above reading, is to present concrete moral guidance for nursing practitioners. The ICN code presupposes the moral competence of nurses because this moral competence is a necessary precondition of their professional status. The presupposition is expressed in the otherwise unarticulated appeal to 'judgment' and 'responsibility'. This is the root ability of the nurse to act morally (and thus to act professionally). The ICN code then merely documents the content of this moral competence, for example, expressing a range of values, such as a commitment to non-discriminatory practice, the respect for confidentiality, and so on, without giving any guidance as to how that general competence is realized in particular situations. This is not the ICN's concern.

This problem can be put in another way. If a code of ethics is to have the objective of guiding everyday practice, then there must be some way of interpreting the very general statements of principle in order to make them applicable to the concrete and in many respects unique problems of everyday practice. This may be illustrated by considering a statement, chosen almost at random, from the Norwegian Nurses' Association's *Ethical Guidelines*: 'The nurse acts to protect the patient/client against illegal or incompetent practice – this includes care and/or treatment as well as research'. The expression of intent here is important and valuable. The patient must indeed be protected from incompetence and unlawful action. Yet the precise meaning of both 'illegal' and 'incompetent' will depend upon the particular context within which they are used. 'Illegality' obviously appeals to the local legal system. More subtly, there will also be local cultural expectations about the degree of competence that can be expected from medical professionals, and also expectations about the circumstances under which those standards might be lowered. There is a gap, therefore, between the general principle and the particular situation to which it must be applied. The interpretation and application of the general principle will require a great deal of knowledge and skill, much of which will be largely taken for granted. For example, the nurse must understand local expectations, and know when a colleague should be excused from full responsibility, perhaps because of illness or excessive work pressure. Similarly, she or he will need to be able to distinguish malicious acts from uncharacteristic blunders, and to respond appropriately. Precisely because of its subtlety and complexity, this taken-for-granted moral knowledge cannot be put into the bold and plain statements of a code.

The problem might be summarized thus: codes, by presenting general principles as guides to action in particular contexts, are in danger of assuming a problem-solving model akin to that found in mathematics. In mathematics, once the general principles of, say, multiplication, have been explained, and given a certain level of mathematical aptitude and competence on the part of the student, then those principles can be applied, unambiguously, to any particular multiplication sum. The claim being made here is that moral problems are of a fundamentally different structure. The complexity of the particular situation is such that no general principle can be unambiguously or incontestably used to resolve it. To begin with, different agents involved in the situation may perceive its moral implications differently. In effect, different people will be attempting to solve different sums. Further, it may be suggested that the idea of a straightforward solution or resolution of moral problems is itself naïve. Few moral problems are worthy of the name if they can be resolved clearly and precisely to everyone's satisfaction, with no residual sense of harm or injustice being felt by any of the parties involved.

This is to suggest that there is an unavoidable gap between the general principles of the code and the particular situation within which a moral problem occurs. Further, this gap poses the key issue for the interpretation of any code. The mathematical analogy used above implies that, unless the principle can be clearly and non-arbitrarily applied to a particular situation, it is meaningless. Codes respond to this problem, and indeed the formulation of the problem according to the mathematical analogy, in various ways. Broad principles can be glossed with commentaries that make them more specific, and that begin to fill out some of the knowledge and skill that is needed to use the general statements. The American code is so structured, and much of the supporting documentation that accompanied the UKCC's code of conduct fulfils a similar role. The recently published *Code of Professional Conduct* (2002) by the new statutory body for UK nursing, the Nursing and Midwifery Council (NMC), also adopts this structure,

but rather than relying on supporting documentation like its predecessor, the commentaries are included in one document. A tradition
of case law may develop, so that it may be recognized that the nurses'
professional body will interpret a principle in a certain way, or within
certain parameters. For example, the NMC's code refers, in the glos-
sary, under 'reasonable', to the Bolam test of reasonable professional
competence (p. 10). Guidance may be given as to how the code is to
be read and interpreted as provided, for example, in the preliminary
material to the Canadian Nurses' Association code. It may be possible
to quantify the practitioner's degree of compliance with certain types
of principle, so that they can be assessed during auditing, which is
a concern of the Australian *Code of Professional Conduct* (ANCI, 1995).
The Norwegian code is not unique in suggesting that the nurse is
expected (according to guideline II.4) to have the 'individual competence', NNA, 1986, p. 3) to assess standards of nursing care, and
thus presumably to understand, possibly after suitable professional
training, how the general principles are to be applied. The issue at stake
here is whether or not any of these attempts at a solution can work,
and the degree to which they presuppose an erroneous mathematical
model of problem-solving in order to work.

The ICN code does not suffer from the same problem of relating the
general to the particular, despite superficial appearances to the contrary, and thus it again provides a clue to understanding the problem of the gap between general and particular. The statements of
principle in the ICN code are indeed highly general. However, if
the objective of the code is a political one rather than an ethical one,
then these general statements do not need to be applied with any
precision to particular situations. If they are read as algorithms for
the solution of moral problems, then, according to the current argument, they are being misread. Rather, it is being suggested that the
ICN code as a whole is to be understood as posing a challenge to
those who are reluctant to take the professional status of the nurse
seriously. It was suggested above that the code must be read as a
response to a question, and the question was formulated as: 'How am
I to present myself, as a professional nurse, to someone who is not
a nurse?' Given this formulation, the challenge can be formulated thus:
'Can you, the outsider, make any sense of my practice as a nurse according to the framework offered by this code?' or 'Can you, for example,
understand how a nurse could have special responsibility for protecting the confidentiality of patient information, or for safeguarding the

patient when threatened by insensitive or inappropriate care from other professionals?' If the code then shapes the nurse's practice, so that it is seen as an expression of her or his professional identity to a hostile outsider, then it cannot be understood as explaining how the nurse could apply concepts of confidentiality or advocacy to her or his practice. It is assumed that the professional nurse can already do that perfectly adequately. In being addressed to outsiders, it is laying down a challenge to them to rethink their preconceptions about nursing. This does not require that the outsider understands nursing as the authors of the code understand it. On the contrary, precisely because the code is an invitation to understand nursing differently, the initial engagement cannot but be a crude realignment of the outsiders' prejudices. The new picture of nursing may still be predominantly shaped within the existing conceptual framework of the respondent. The code will have served its initial purpose if it has begun to win nursing more serious consideration. The precise details of that serious consideration will no doubt be articulated, at the national or local level, much later. In summary, this is to suggest that the ICN code is the focus of a debate, and not the source of instruction and guidance.

If the ICN codes' objectives are different from those of the national codes, then, *prima facie*, they make poor models, and passages transferred verbatim to the national codes will be more or less subtly changed in meaning. It may be noted, however, that certain codes, despite their overt statement of objectives, may still be part of the political struggle to professional status for nursing. Thus the Finnish code concludes with the following exhortation:

> Nurses are responsible for the expertise of their profession. They are active in developing a core of professional knowledge, and they enhance nursing education and the scientific basis of nursing. The enhancement of nursing expertise should be reflected in the improved well-being of the population. (FFN, 1997, p. 1)

Crucially, this code (and others like it) serves to shift the issue of professionalization away from a core moral expertise and towards a technical or scientific expertise. The ethical status of this passage is only partially reinstated by the final clause, and the appeal to the wellbeing of the population. The code thus breaks from its ICN model in this crucial and yet problematic respect. While the ICN presupposes ethical competence, and uses that as the basic of professionalization, the Finnish code sees ethical competence as something yet to be acquired and thus gives guidance to its readers on ethical practice and decision-making. In shifting the issue of professionalization, the code offers a different understanding of what the professional nurse is. The nurse fulfils an objective or has a 'mission' similar to that stated by the ICN, namely 'to promote and maintain the health of the population, prevent illness, and alleviate suffering', but does so primarily through technical expertise, not moral judgement. It may then be argued that the Finnish code, like the ICN code, is posing a challenge to the unsympathetic outsider, but now asks if that outsider can come to understand nursing as a technical profession. This then leaves the status of the overtly moral elements of the code ambiguous, for they have been largely borrowed from the ICN code, and yet now as problems needing guidance, rather than as resources enabling professionalization. Because the outsider is not asked to understand nursing in ethical terms, the gap between the particular moral situation and general moral statement is left unbridged.

To look at this another way, the Finnish code may be seen to have set up a dichotomy between politics and ethics. The political aspect of the code centres upon the self-presentation of the nurse to the outsider, and leads to the challenge to understand nursing as a profession; the ethical centres on the regulation of the nurse's practice. The ICN code does not invoke this dichotomy, as the ethical is presupposed as the ground of the political. Thus the ICN code may be offering a richer and more plausible model of ethics.

It has been argued that the overtly ethical objective of various national codes, to guide everyday practice, leads to the problem of bridging the gap between general principle and a particular situation. A number of responses to that problem were noted above, all working, to some significant degree, with a mathematical analogy of problem-solving. It has been suggested here that these responses will not work. One solution offered, and that most literally working within a mathematical model, was to quantify the degree of compliance with standards, in order to allow auditing. Yet quantification will work only in certain cases, for example, in providing precise standards for in-service training. The contention here, however, is that moral problems are distinctive not least in the recognition that they cannot be quantified.

To provide further textual glosses on a bold statement may indeed help to make it more concrete, but glosses and interpretative statements can never capture the uniqueness of every concrete moral problem. Thus the practitioner must, at some level, still have to use her or his judgement, drawing on taken-for-granted knowledge of the local environment and how to act effectively within it in order to cope with a particular problem. Yet glosses begin to have a positive role, and begin to approach the conception of ethics that is being advocated, in so far as they say something unexpected. For example, in explicating the principle that, 'The nurse in all professional relationships, practices with compassion and respect for the inherent dignity, worth and uniqueness of every individual, unrestricted by considerations of social or economic status, personal attributes, or the nature of health problems', the American code comments on care of the dying at considerable length in the interpretative statements emphasizing compassion, patient autonomy and self-determination as the basis for informed consent, the right to accurate information and the importance of support in decision-making.

The interpretative statements may be criticized for being unnecessarily verbose, but they do something important by making the reader aware, for example, that death is a moral problem and, indeed, a complex one that will not submit to easy solution. The banal statements that make up the principles of the American, and many other, codes pose the problem of why a professional, possessed of the ICN's 'judgment' and 'responsibility', should need to be instructed in such common-sense maxims. In contrast, some points of commentary can break through the complacency of common sense, and challenge the reader to see a moral problem where perhaps otherwise it would have eluded her or him. Again, the gap between general and particular is bridged, not through the assumption of a mathematical model, and the further refinement of the algorithm needed to solve the problem, but rather by challenging the reader to see and interpret the world differently. The ethics lies in the recognition of the problem, not in its solution.

An appeal to case law or examples may serve to invoke the uniqueness of the situation. Section 14 of the UKCC's *Guidelines for Professional Practice* (1996), which was itself a substantial commentary on the UKCC *Code of Professional Conduct*), offered three examples of '[h]ow circumstances can affect your duty of care'. The examples involve the manner in which a 'skilled adult intensive care nurse' will respond to a patient suffering a cardiac arrest within an intensive care unit, a women giving birth in a hospital corridor, and an injured person at the scene of a traffic accident (UKCC, 1996, p. 5). Precisely because of their concreteness, the examples dramatize the moral problem. They work less because they attempt to bring general principles down to the particular situation, and more because they force the reader to reflect upon the everyday knowledge and skills to judge and make sense of a situation, and one's place within it, that are fundamental to ethical practice. To make sense of the example requires the reader to draw upon precisely those skills and that knowledge which they would use in a real situation. It is precisely these skills that were introduced above, with respect to the Norwegian code's concern with illegality and competence.

The solution posed at the centre of the Norwegian code, that the nurse has the individual competence and other resources to assess standards, leads to the most profound paradox. The principles of the Norwegian code are unremarkable, again to the point of banality. A paradox therefore arises because, on the one hand, the nurse appears to need to be told that, for example, patient or client rights must be safeguarded 'as regards use of confidential information', and on the other, the nurse is attributed a significant degree of individual moral competence, even if this is merely the competence of knowing when and how to seek advice from elsewhere. If the Norwegian code is addressed primarily to nurses, rather than to the presentation of the idea of professional nursing to outsiders, then it is left with the paradox that nurses are at once morally naïve and morally sophisticated. The code therefore either tells the morally competent nurse what she or he already knows, or leaves the morally incompetent nurse as unenlightened as ever.

The above analysis has therefore suggested that some form of moral competence is a precondition for reading and understanding a code of general principles. However, this competence is not akin to that of the mathematician, for it does not entail the ability to apply general algorithmic principles to the solution of well-defined and particular problems. Consideration of the bridging tactics of examples and glosses has begun to suggest that moral competence lies, not in the application of general principles, but in the ability to experience a situation as morally problematic. This understanding of moral competence will be further elucidated, in the next section of this chapter, through consideration of two further codes, that of the Canadian Nurses' Association (1997) and the *Ethical Guidelines and Principles of Practice for Catholic Nursing and Midwifery Personnel* (CICIAMS, 1988).

A source for education and reflection

The Canadian Nurses' Association's code, adopted in 1985 and revised in 1997, is one of the few national codes that breaks significantly and explicitly from the ICN model (Yeo, 1991, pp. 222–237). The code offers objectives for nursing that are not dissimilar to the ICN model, such as: 'Nurses value health and well-being and assist persons to achieve their optimum level of health in situations of normal health, illness, injury or in the process of dying' (CNA, 1997, p. 6). The inter-relationship of nursing and moral competence is explicitly stated: 'Ethical reflection and judgment are required to determine how a particular value or responsibility applies in a particular nursing context' (p. 4). The main part of the code is made up of a set of general moral principles or 'values' and their interpretation as 'standards'. There is, however, also significant material on the nature of ethics, and the way in which a code should be used, and thus on the way in which moral competence is to be understood and developed. In this context, in addition to the provision of guidance for everyday practice, the code is also given the following justification:

> The Code of Ethics for registered Nurses gives guidance for decision making concerning ethical matters, serves as a means for self-evaluation and reflection regarding ethical nursing practice and provides a basis for peer review initiatives. The code not only educates nurses about their ethical responsibilities, but also informs other health care professionals and members of the public about the moral commitments expected of nurses. (CNA, 1997, p. 1)

Other codes may present themselves, perhaps incidentally, as resources for reflection and self-evaluation; the Canadian code is distinctive in being concerned with the sort of conditions that must be fulfilled in order to facilitate this reflection. Crucially, it recognizes that moral reflection may, and under certain circumstances must, entail rational discussion with others.

The code distinguishes 'ethical violations' from 'ethical dilemmas'. The former 'involve the neglect of moral obligation', and the example of failure to care for a patient simply through the desire to avoid personal inconvenience is given. The latter 'arise when ethical reasons both for and against a particular course of action are present'. It may be suggested that the majority of codes of nursing ethics, precisely in the banality of what they say, concern themselves with ethical violations.

These are straightforward cases where all but the most morally insensitive would recognize the problem, and thus where moral reflection, for example on the principles of the code, would itself be largely futile as it could do little more than rehearse that which is self-evident. The idea of an ethical dilemma opens up a distinctive way of understanding ethical competence. The Canadian code glosses it as follows:

> There is room within the profession of nursing for disagreement among nurses about the relative weight of different ethical values and principles. More than one proposed intervention might be ethical and reflective of good practice. Discussion is extremely helpful in the resolution of ethical issues. (CNA, 1997, p. 4)

On this account, there must be situations in which the moral problem is understood differently by the different parties involved and where no resolution is self-evidently correct. Moral competence, and indeed moral reflection, therefore entails an openness towards, and a tolerance of, the views of others.

The Canadian code explicitly says little more about the problem of ethical dilemmas. It is perhaps not an exaggeration to say that they represent an innovation in professional ethics that is not easily contained within the conventions of codes. A number of 'limitations' are noted where exceptional circumstances entail that moral principles cannot be applied in the usual way. This important category is perhaps under-used, for it serves to illustrate much about the complexity of moral judgement.[8] The code implicitly goes beyond this, for both of its categories of 'values' and 'standards' break, to some degree, from the traditional presentation of principles and interpretative statements. The standards work best when, like the interpretative statements in the American code, they serve to challenge taken-for-granted understandings of the moral dimensions of a situation. An example will suffice. It glosses '[n]urses value and advocate the dignity and self-respect of human beings', before going on to suggest, for example, that nurses respect the bodily privacy of clients when care is given. This example challenges because it transfigures the cliché of 'dignity' into the more concrete language of privacy. This potentially opens up for reflection, not simply a new aspect of a moral problem, but also a new way of talking morally.

The code makes a number of comments on 'values' and claims that it is 'organized around seven primary values that are central to ethical nursing' (p. 3). From this it may be suggested that the values articulate what it means to be a nurse. In effect, we return to the questions that motivated the ICN code. Two formulations of the question were given. The first, provisional, version ran as follows: 'What, morally, is entailed in being a nurse; or how am I to understand myself, morally, as a nurse?' The second formulation was this: 'How am I to present myself, as a professional nurse, to someone who is not a nurse?'

The shift from the first question to the second occurred once it was recognized that the ICN's objectives were political, rather than ethical. It may be suggested that the Canadian code has begun, not simply to find a way in which to answer the first question, but, more precisely, to offer a framework within which the nurse can present her or his own answer. Thus the Canadian code is a genuinely ethical code. The issue of professionalization is not wholly alien to the Canadian code, but by making the problematic nature of ethical dilemmas its core, and thus in dispensing largely with the mathematical model of problem-solving, it has begun to indicate that there is a fundamental relationship between the way in which the nurse understands her or himself as a moral being, and the way in which she or he understands a moral problem. This final claim might be substantiated to some degree through an analysis of the CICIAMS code.

This code of guidelines and principles of practice for nursing and midwifery, is presented in a largely orthodox structure of boldly stated principles. Yet the distinctiveness of the code is apparent at a number of points. First, ethical problems are seen to emerge from a changing social, cultural and technological context,[9] rather than from that which is routine. Second, the Catholic nurse's practice is grounded in Christian principles[10] and Christian vision.[11] This leads to onerous demands:

> (3.3) All persons must always act according to their conscience. No one should be forced to act contrary to their religious, ethical or moral convictions. International law recognises the right to Conscientious objection. Where this right is not specifically recognised in legislation or de facto, Catholic Nurses have the duty to work to change that situation through the institutions and organisations that represent them. (CICIAMS, 1988, p. 3)

This contrasts markedly with the more typical article on conscientious objection found in the NMC *Code of Professional Conduct* (2002):

> 2.5 You must report to a relevant person or authority, at the earliest possible time, any conscientious objection that may be relevant to your professional practice. You must continue to provide care to the best of your ability until alternative arrangements are implemented. (p. 4)

Here, then, is the core distinction between the Catholic code and other more traditional codes. Traditional codes, unwittingly echoing the politics of the ICN, subordinate the personal resources and characteristic of the nurse to her or his professional status. The nurse must understand her or himself primarily as a professional nurse. The Catholic code places the nurse's existence as a Catholic before professional status. The code therefore responds to the question: 'What, as a Catholic, is entailed in being a nurse?'; or 'How am I to understand myself, as a Catholic, as a nurse?' To understand oneself as a Catholic is, according to the presentation of this code, to understand ethical problems in a distinctive way, a way that breaks from the orthodox ICN framework. The consequence of this is that one may disagree with the Catholic code, for example, in its resistance to euthanasia, or its insistence on helping patients to die according to their belief, but precisely in disagreeing you are challenged to ask yourself why, and thus to articulate, not simply the reasons for this disagreement, but more profoundly the kind of person you are, and how that personal and moral identity influences your nursing practice.

Conclusion

A slightly random selection of codes has been considered. Different codes have different objectives and present moral issues with greater or lesser insight. It has been suggested that the ICN code is effective only if it is understood as politically situated in the struggle to professionalize nursing. The nurse is thus encouraged to understand her or himself as a beleaguered professional. Moral competence is a precondition of that professionalism, and ethical problems, in large part, focus on anything that may threaten that professional autonomy. A misreading of the 1973 ICN code as a set of practice guidelines leads to documents such as the Norwegian or Finnish codes. Precisely by insisting on banal or commonly accepted principles, the codes paradoxically imply that the person, as a person rather than as a nurse, has no worthwhile moral competence, with the perceived threat of conscientious objection being the apogee of this line of thought. The paradox lies in the failure to bridge the gap between general principle and particular situation without reliance on the practitioner's moral competence, expressed, for example, as 'judgement'. This paradox must lead to the ineffectiveness of the codes as moral documents. Without the practitioner's prior moral knowledge, they are useless. Yet, if the practitioner is already morally competent, then he or she will learn nothing from these codes.

It has therefore been suggested that only those codes that challenge and indeed disturb the reader can be effective. This is to argue that the image of a professional nurse that the ICN code places before those who are unsympathetic to professional nursing must be transformed into explicitly moral images. The primary purpose of this moral image is not to challenge the outsider, but to challenge the nurse her- or himself. Only then can the nurse confidently present this self-understanding to outsiders.

The Catholic code draws upon what it means to be a Catholic in order to challenge our understanding of what it is to be a nurse. The Canadian code, perhaps less radically, appeals to the rationality and liberality of the practitioner. Moral competence lies, not in the ability to solve moral problems like mathematical sums, but rather in being able to recognize the complexity, tragedy and conflict of moral dilemmas, and to be able to struggle, alone or preferably though discussion with others, to make as much sense of them as possible. Ultimately, moral competence allows one to do something, and what precisely one does depends on the understanding of what it means to be a professional nurse in that unique situation.

Notes

1. The term 'hermeneutics' refers to the theory of interpretation. This chapter is therefore primarily concerned with the way in which meaning may be extracted from and attributed to codes.

2. It may be noted that this chapter does not attempt a systematic or exhaustive overview of nursing codes. While it is hoped that the codes to which reference is made are broadly representative, they have largely been chosen in so far as they make possible the illustration and development of a specific point of argument or analysis.

3. A remark on the methodology of this reading may be appropriate. The following readings are based on a close attention to the texts of codes themselves, with little or no attempt to explore the actual social and cultural conditions within which they were written or within which they are read. Conclusions about these conditions are derived from attempts to produce as consistent a reading of the codes as possible, and specifically to deal with apparent weaknesses within them.

4. It may thus be noted that the 1953 ICN code begins with the claim that 'Professional nurses *minister* to the sick' (italics added). Similarly, the Florence Nightingale pledge describes nursing as a calling. The pledge refers to the need to respect patient confidentiality, but also asserts that 'With loyalty will I endeavour to aid the physician in his work, and devote myself to the welfare of those committed to my care' (Davis and Aroskar, 1978, pp. 8f).

5. 'The nurse maintains the highest standards of nursing care possible within the reality of a specific situation...The nurse...participates in establishing and maintaining equitable social and economic working conditions.'

6. 'The nurse uses judgment in relation to individual competence when accepting and delegating responsibilities.'

7. 'The nurse takes appropriate action to safeguard the individual when his care is endangered by a co-worker or any other person.'

8. Something similar may be noted with respect the material provided by the UKCC: '... *with a view to removal from the register...* '? documents situations under which a nurse can be proven to have been culpable of misconduct, and yet should not have their professional registration removed. These include the incident being isolated and uncharacteristic; it was influenced by overwhelming personal problems, now resolved; it was an error of judgement rather than a culpable act (section 37). Despite the quasi-legal status of this, and other UKCC documents, it does serve to invoke the subtlety with which a genuine moral competence must respond to the particular situation, and does so far more effectively than in any other UKCC publication.

9. For example (from 0.2): 'The concept of mankind conveyed and imposed by the media, imperceptibly alters the image man has of himself and health.'

10. '(1.1) For the Catholic Nurse the services of the human race is rooted in Loving Kindness which stems from God.'

11. 'When in contact with suffering, the Nurses draw inspiration from the Christian vision of the paschal mystery of Christ the Saviour, so they carry out a true Ministry, recognised by the Church, in the service of life and health.' The use of 'Ministry' can of course be compared to its (metaphorical) use in the 1953 ICN code.

References

American Nurses' Association (2001) *Code for Nurses*, Kansas: ANA.
Australian Nursing Council Incorporated (1995) *Code of Professional Conduct for Nurses in Australia*, Melbourne: ANCI.

Callahan, J.C. (ed.) (1988) *Ethical Issues in Professional Life*, Oxford: Oxford University Press.

Canadian Nurses' Association (1997) *Code of Ethics for Registered Nurses*, Ottawa: CNA.

CICIAMS (International Catholic Committee of Nurses and Medico-Social Assistants) (1988) *Ethical Guidelines and Principles of Practice for Catholic Nursing and Midwifery Personnel*, Brussels: CICIAMS.

Davis, A. and Aroskar, M.A. (1978) *Ethical Dilemmas and Nursing Practice*, New York: Appleton-Century-Crofts.

Finnish Federation of Nurses (1997) *Ethical Guidelines for Nurses*, Helsinki: FFA.

ICN (International Council of Nurses) (1973) *Code for Nurses: Ethical Concepts Applied to Nursing*, Geneva: ICN.

MacIntryre, A. (1981) *After Virtue*, London: Duckworth.

NMC (Nursing and Midwifery Council) *Code of Professional Conduct*, London: NMC.

Norwegian Nurse's Association (1986) *Ethical Guidelines for Nurses* (English translation), Oslo: NNA.

United Kingdom Central Council for Nursing, Midwifery and Health Visiting (1990) '...*with a view to removal from the register*...'? London: UKCC.

United Kingdom Central Council for Nursing, Midwifery and Health Visiting (1992) *Code of Professional Conduct*, London: UKCC.

United Kingdom Central Council for Nursing, Midwifery and Health Visiting (1996) *Guidelines of Professional Practice*, London: UKCC.

Yeo, M. (1991) *Concepts and Cases in Nursing Ethics*, Peterborough, Ontario: Broadview Press.

10

Professional Self-Regulation in Nursing

Reg Pyne

Introduction

Those who, like me, received their education and training to enter the nursing profession in the United Kingdom and have, for all or most of their professional career, practised in the same country, have a tendency to regard the professional regulatory systems that prevail in their country of original qualification as natural and assume that they are universal. I imagine that, in this respect, nurses in other countries are prone to make the same assumptions. It can come as something of a surprise to find that this is not true. I personally experienced that feeling of surprise in the 1970s when, having been awarded a Council of Europe Medical Fellowship for the express purpose of studying the means by which, and manner in which, the health professions generally, and my own profession of nursing in particular, were regulated in a range of European countries, I travelled to those countries with my preconceived ideas.

The fact that I had prepared a submission to undertake this study and subsequently convinced an impressive interview panel that I was deserving of the award can be taken as an indication that I knew or suspected that there were differences, and that these differences might take on greater significance when the first directive concerning the 'general care nurse' became operative in the European Community as it was composed in the 1970s. I certainly knew more than the average UK registered nurse about the subject, since I was at the time a senior member of staff of my own country's nursing regulatory body, frequently engaged in evaluating applications for registration from persons whose original registration was obtained in a country outside the United Kingdom. Another of my duties was to verify, for comparable registration bodies in other countries, the registration and current good standing of nurses with original registration in the UK who wished to register with them as a prelude to professional practice. But 'Freedom of Movement' within the countries of the European Community for a very large number of qualified nurses was about to come over the horizon, and it seemed wise to try to enhance my knowledge, draw some conclusions and share my findings.

Summary

The content of this chapter is based on my experiences while undertaking the Fellowship described above, my work as an officer of two regulatory bodies in the UK and latterly as a consultant for the International Council of Nurses (ICN).

The chapter begins with some brief comments about nurse regulation in Europe, followed by a section exploring the development of professional regulation in the UK. It moves on to examine the challenges to professional regulation before considering the essential requirements of any professional regulatory system.

The remainder of the chapter is concerned with examining five key principles which should underpin professional regulation. These are: identifying the purpose of the regulation; clarifying the essential elements of a regulatory system; considering who the interested parties are and how they should be involved; recognizing any hazards which must be avoided and ensuring that the system is both fair and just.

The chapter concludes by challenging nurses to address whether their regulatory systems are as robust as they ought to be.

The 1970s and nursing registration in Europe

I was, at the time, familiar with a system by which the nursing profession in my own country was regulated by an organization (then the General Nursing Council for England and Wales, or GNCEW) in which nurses elected by their fellow practitioners filled 22 of the 42 member places. Of the remainder, all of whom were appointed by the government ministers with responsibility for health, more than half were also nurses, the remainder being composed of medical practitioners, senior managers in the health services and persons with specialist educational experience. The membership included not even one person who had been appointed for the purpose of bringing an explicit lay or consumer view to the Council's deliberations and decision-making, yet the claim made for the whole regulatory activity, though never explicitly stated in the law that established the Council, was that of protection of the public.

In all of these respects the structure of the Nursing Council mirrored other organizations established under various Acts of Parliament for the medical and dental professions and a number of other occupational groups in the health field. This was the system that, at that time, I assumed, allowing for minor variations, to be the norm. How surprised I was soon to be! As I visited and met key people in government health departments, professional membership organizations, trades unions and places where nurses worked around Europe, and as I supplemented this with correspondence with equivalent people in a number of other European countries that I was not able to visit, I quickly found that what I regarded as standard was not standard at all. Although the British system had been copied and implemented with some variations in many countries of the former British Empire, the only other European country with a system that bore any substantial similarity to it was the Republic of Ireland, but that was not to say it was exactly the same.

In the system I knew, the nurse members of the Council, although operating within the framework of government legislation, played the dominant role in making decisions about the form and content of nursing education and training and the qualifying examinations and assessments that were a prelude to entry to professional practice as a registered nurse. They formed a substantial majority in the Council that employed experienced nurse educators to inspect nurse training schools and recommend that they either retain or lose that role. Nurses also composed a majority of the Council members who served on what was then the Disciplinary Committee, which met to hear evidence concerning alleged misconduct and exercised the power to remove persons from the register for what was judged to be 'professional misconduct', thereby preventing them from practising in their chosen profession. In this way the Council, operating as almost a representative body for the profession, was able to exercise fairly strict control over the content of education and training, who could gain access to it, the places in which it could be provided, the standard required to obtain the professional qualification that was a prerequisite to admission to the register, and the opportunity to continue in practice.

What I found from my Fellowship studies was that the norm for other countries varied from the absence of any recognizable system of professional regulation, to direct regulation by an arm of the relevant government department, usually the Ministry of Health, with a loose form of institutional regulation operated mainly by employers falling somewhere between the two. In some countries, it seemed to me that there was very little opportunity for nurses to exercise even a modest influence on the content of their education and training programmes, and certainly no prospect of them having the dominant say. The variation was enormous, as was the impact of the regulatory systems with nurse involvement where that did exist. Indeed, it was clear that in some countries the descriptive term 'professional self-regulation' had no place, since nurses either played no part or had only a minority voice in matters related to the regulation of their profession.

The development of professional regulation in the United Kingdom

Reverting briefly to the system that existed in the United Kingdom in the 1970s, it was, as stated, a similar model to that provided for other occupational groups regarded as 'professions' within the health sector. The pattern had been set in the middle of the nineteenth century by the establishment of the General Medical Council as a means of determining which of the several factions then practising 'medicine' were to be regarded as the legally recognized definitive practitioners, leaving those outside the fold as 'quacks'. Expectations had been expressed, not least by one of the General Medical Council's early Presidents, that similar councils for other groups, particularly nurses, would soon be established. Although there was much pressure for this to happen, it was not until the early years of the twentieth century that any new legislation to this effect was passed by the British Parliament. A 'Board' to regulate the profession of midwifery was established by a law of 1902. This, however, was to remain largely dominated by medical practitioners until its replacement in 1983. The General Nursing Council was born as a result of the Nurses' Registration Act of 1919. In this case, although elected practising nurses composed only a small minority of the membership in the early years, this changed over time to the small elected majority situation applying in the 1970s, a further number of nurses being added through the government appointment process. It has to recognized, however, that although the structure and system provided for nurses was something of an imitation of the medical profession's regulatory system, it was a relatively pale imitation, as the Nursing Council was never given the position of power in their relation to the government that the Medical Council had enjoyed for so long.

Challenges to professional regulation

During the last quarter of the twentieth century and into the twenty-first, a great deal has changed in many countries of the world in respect of the regulation of the health professions, and the UK has not been immune from this. Even where the regulatory structures have continued in basically similar form, they have been more exposed to challenge and questioning than ever before. A number of countries – not least the UK – have experienced periods with governments in power actively pursuing a deregulation agenda, and the health professions have been in the sights of those with reforming zeal in this direction. In many cases the interference experienced was more by way of nibbling away at the powers of the regulatory bodies than their removal or outright reform, but clearly the end of that particular chapter has yet to be written in many countries.

Coincident with challenge from governmental sources, there has been something still more significant – the emergence of 'grassroots' challenge. During that same period of time, many members of the public developed higher expectations of members of the health professions, are now less deferential to members of those professions, and are better informed about issues that affect their lives than ever before. Is it any surprise that they now challenge and question the professionals more often and from a basis of knowledge? This is also an age in which more health care and treatment than ever before is delivered by members of different professions, often with overlapping scopes of practice, working together in teams, their individual accountability supplemented by a corporate accountability. Alert members of the public are aware of this, and are, with increasing frequency, asking if it really makes sense, in the early years of the twenty-first century, to continue to adhere to what is essentially a nineteenth-century model of professional regulation. Nurses, like members of other health professions, including medicine, need to construct an appropriate and positive 'public interest' response to this new situation.

The role of the ICN

Fortunately, nursing, both at national level in some countries and particularly at international level through the ICN, has been active in this area, not as a means of expressing self-interest and defending its position, but rather with the intention of constructing systems of regulation that genuinely address the public interest. The ICN took a lead in this respect in 1985 when it produced and published its first position statement on professional regulation. It was my privilege, when a decision was taken to review that statement with a view to revision in 1996, to be engaged by ICN as the consultant for the project. This enabled me to undertake a massive literature search identifying the challenges to professional regulation that were emerging in many countries of the world and to prepare detailed papers for consideration by the internationally representative expert group assembled to work with me in the second phase. As a result of this work, the conclusion reached was that although the existing twelve principles remained valid, in order to address the emergent challenges and to recommend a framework appropriate to the beginning of a new century, each needed to be supported by fresh narrative and clearly stated policy objectives. The new text resulting from this work was published by ICN in September 1997 under the title *International Council of Nurses on Regulation: Toward 21st Century Models* (ICN, 1997).

With that outline model available as a template against which to construct future systems, and now that we have entered that new century, there seems little point in excessive analysis of the past or even study of the present. Recognizing the need to look forward and assist the development of appropriate models of professional regulation in all countries, whether they currently have a sophisticated system in operation or not, and given my unsurprising support for the ICN position statement that I helped to construct, much of the rest of this chapter argues a case with great similarities to that seminal text.

In the opening passages of the text, ICN, having first described 'regulation' as a means by which order, consistency and control can be brought to a profession and its practice, sets down the 'rationale' for the construction of the document, incorporating this statement of intent:

> Health is a vital social asset; 'Health for All' (WHO, 1995) is a global objective. The nursing profession intends to offer its utmost to this worldwide social purpose. Fulfilling this promise calls for influencing and responding to changing health needs and priorities, and developing and mobilising the fullest potential of the profession. (ICN, 1997, p. 1)

The resolution by which ICN approved and launched the new position statement makes clear its conclusion that 'a system of governance for the profession' must be constructed around four key objectives. These, in effect, are:

> systems that allow and encourage personal and professional growth in order to achieve high standards of practice;

> authority for nurses to practise to the full extent of their competence and skill;

> engagement of the profession in the development of public policy, allied to a means of accountability to the public for its individual and corporate performance; and

> recognition of the contributions of the profession reflected in the appropriate remuneration of its members and their opportunities to develop. (ICN, 1997, p. 2)

Not everyone will accept that the last of these objectives is a role for the body charged with regulation; those who take a different view usually regard it as being better handled by other means and through a parallel process. It is, however, difficult to argue with the other objectives if the intent is to be honoured. Significantly, it is not the ICN position that these objectives can only be achieved by a single system model that should be applied in all countries.

While the parts of the text that state ICN's reasoning and resolve are important, still more important to those developing a system of professional regulation or reviewing an existing system are the sections that set out the principles on which such a system should be founded, together with the constructive narrative that supports them. The document states twelve principles, which I have reduced to five essential questions to which responses must be provided. These are:

- What is the purpose of a system of professional regulation?
- What are the essential elements of the design of such a system?
- Who are the interested parties and how should they be involved?
- What hazards must be avoided?
- How do you ensure fairness, justice and opportunities for those regulated?

What is the purpose of a system of regulation?

The first question ICN tackles head on. The first principle states unequivocally that regulation should be directed towards an explicit purpose. This may seem to be so obvious as to be unnecessary. I contend that it is needed, and is appropriately stated first. Even where (as in the UK) the regulatory organization is established by a separate Act of Parliament, it is rare to find the explicit purpose described. ICN has surely been right to recommend that it be stated, not least because there is much evidence of a rising tide of informed public dissatisfaction with the way in which some regulatory bodies have conducted their affairs. The opinion that they have been self-serving rather than concentrating on addressing the public interest has frequently been expressed in recent years. So the principle is reinforced by the firm statement that 'The overriding purpose of the statutory regulation of nursing is that of service to and protection of the public.' Further reinforcement comes with this:

> Benefits to the profession and individual practitioners are secondary and, although they can be significant, do not of themselves provide justification for statutory regulation. They may receive appropriate attention through other regulatory processes but the public interest must not be compromised as a result. (ICN, 1997, cited in Pyne, 1998, pp. 248–249)

To its credit, ICN has recognized that, in order to achieve this position, two things are essential. First, the organization responsible for regulating the profession must be innovative rather than passive. Second, individual practitioners must 'adopt a dynamic approach to their role, striving to achieve their full potential in the service of the public and accepting responsibility to critically reappraise their practice as health care changes' (ibid.).

Risking the criticism of those who might say it is another statement of the obvious, the ICN text reinforces the first contention with the next principle – 'Since the overriding purpose of statutory regulation is service to and protection of the public, the regulatory system should be designed to satisfy this intent in a comprehensive manner' (ibid.). This principle is also developed in an unequivocal manner, focusing attention on both the individual practitioner and the settings in which they practice.

Of the former it is stated as essential that the individual practitioner:

[a] recognise the importance of maintaining and improving their knowledge, skills, ethical awareness and competence throughout professional life; [b] use all opportunities to improve the quality and standard of nursing care; and [c] accept this responsibility as an integral part of their personal accountability for professional practice. (Ibid.)

But the individual practitioner cannot do it all alone, so the following key statement is made related to practice settings: 'practice settings are supportive of practitioners, allowing practice to develop and flourish' (ibid.). And that, of course means that standards of education must be relevant to now and not some past practice age, that examinations and any other assessment measures must relate to those standards, and that the standards for practice must be subject to periodical critical review to ensure that they remain valid in changing circumstances.

What are the essential elements of the design of a regulatory system?

ICN's response to this question comes largely through the third and fourth principles and their supportive narrative. Once again they proclaim the need for a firm foundation associated with the need to keep abreast of changes in practice. I endorse the conclusions that are drawn and contend that they address the system design question appropriately.

The third principle states the case for clear definitions of professional scope and accountability. That statement, if applied in a narrow mechanistic manner, defining professional practice around a list of permitted tasks, would be disastrous. It is saved from that, however, by the emphasis placed on the fact that 'the nurse is both responsible and accountable for the breadth of nursing practice, involving others where this is considered appropriate'. (ICN, 1997, cited in Pyne, 1998, pp. 249–250)

That applies equally to delegation to another suitably supervised person or to the involvement of a specialist whose knowledge and competence can best deliver the care required in a particular situation.

As for defining 'professional scope', it would be foolish of me to try to improve on the excellent statement found in the narrative as follows:

> ICN's clear preference, and therefore its strong recommendation, is that legislation adopt a flexible approach to 'scope of practice' issues. ICN recognises and accepts that benefits in service delivery can result from overlapping scopes of practice among different health professions and that a dynamic approach to professional practice will enable greater public service result. (ICN, 1997, cited in Pyne, 1998, p. 250)

Historically far too many regulatory systems prevented practitioners from developing their role and consequently failed to allow them to serve the public to their full capacity. If that was ever appropriate (which is unlikely), it is no longer the case. Inappropriately restrictive legislation hampers professional practice and is contrary to the genuine public interest.

The second part of the response to the 'essential elements' question is that 'it should promote the fullest development of the profession commensurate with its potential social contribution' (ibid.). So again the case against stagnation and for development emerges. That attitude, and the commensurate action, is required from both nurses as individuals and the organization charged with the regulatory function. As individuals, nurses must develop their capacity to meet new challenges, be active as citizens and attempt to influence the policy debates that affect the context of their professional practice, as well as being agents of positive change rather than victims of change that is planned and imposed by others. But the organizations that bear the responsibility for regulation have responsibilities in this area as well. While it is absolutely right for them to help set out the platform for professional practice through published codes, guidelines and standards documents, they fail those same people completely if they are silent about the broad areas of health policy and the context in which nurses have to practise. Whether they are, in effect, an arm of a government health department, or a separate organization charged in law with regulatory responsibilities, it is essential that they engage at a high level in the sort of dialogue that makes clear the realities of the context of professional practice.

Who are the interested parties and how should they be involved?

The answer to this question must obviously start with 'the public', since it is their interests rather than those of the profession that the whole regulatory process is intended to serve. Traditionally the direct involvement of people who bring a genuinely 'lay' perspective as representatives of the public interest has been extremely limited, if indeed it has existed at all. Other than in those societies where this would not be consistent with local conventions or, for some other valid reason it is not yet possible, it must now be regarded as right to involve public representatives to the maximum degree possible. Failure to do so is paternalistic and offensive.

In many countries (not least my own), where the regulatory bodies have been subjected to increasing levels of challenge and criticism for their perceived failures or perverse decisions that have reinforced the 'self-serving' image, the percentage of lay or public members has been steadily increased. However, this remained a minority of the membership until the advent of the Nursing and Midwifery Council (NMC) in 2002, whose membership consists of 11 lay and 12 professional, and it is sometimes necessary to wonder what it is that the professions are afraid of.

Just as the public are major stakeholders, so also is the government of the country. At the very minimum their role must be to put in place the appropriate legislation and to review and revise it as and when necessary. In addition it is incumbent on the government, either directly or by delegation, to develop and operate the law that regulates education for practice, practice itself, in an enabling rather than limiting way, and the employment setting.

Reference to the employment setting opens up the question of the role of employers in the total process of regulation. Since most nurses do not work in independent practice, the employers provide the practice setting for the vast majority of them. They need, therefore, to be aware of the standards promoted by the profession's regulatory body, and there seems no good reason why some representatives of employers should not be directly involved in its work. This would help to ensure that in developing their institutional standards, employers generally achieve consistency with those promoted by the regulatory body, thereby avoiding the risk of conflict for individual practitioners.

It seems self-evident that employers will want nurses to provide the best possible care and best outcomes for their patients and they normally recognize that this is best achieved when the environment enables nurses to practise competently and ethically.

Given the fact that an increasing amount of care and treatment is delivered by practitioners from different health professions working together in teams, it seems equally logical that while a situation is perpetuated of separate regulatory bodies for medicine, nursing and other professions, some membership places in those bodies should be filled by the other professions. It is clearly not in the public interest for any single profession to be unchallenged in its regulatory processes and standards, to dominate other professions, or to develop in isolation when shared practice is the order of the day. The conclusion I have reached and believe to be logical is that a united system of professional regulation is becoming harder to resist. I have argued this in *Consumer Policy Review* (Pyne, 2000), and also find support in a recent UK publication from the National Consumer Council (NCC, 1999). The latter document, *Self-Regulation of Professionals in Health Care*, describes the present position in the UK as 'a patchwork of varying arrangements for different professions, differences in regulation between public and independent sectors and legislation governing many regulatory bodies which has not caught up with changes in public demand or with current health practice' (p. 1). It would not be wise to ignore this criticism at a time when the consumer voice is becoming ever more strident and articulate. I suspect that much the same criticism could be levelled at the systems of regulation currently in operation in many other countries.

Finally, the profession must also be numbered among the stakeholders in the activity of regulation. Nursing needs to be vigilant in monitoring the effectiveness of existing systems of regulation and promoting positive change. It should not be regarded as acceptable for the profession to sit back, wait for proposals from elsewhere, and then react. Just as it is right and proper to involve the other parties mentioned and join with them in the formal and informal processes of professional regulation, it is also right for the profession to set the pace and take a lead in respect of its own governance. The most essential element is that the profession demonstrates its sensitivity to the public interest. This more than anything will generate understanding and support for the developments in practice that nurses, individually and collectively, wish to promote. This contention finds reinforcement in the ICN text which states of the profession, 'It must promote vigorously that component of professional regulation which the individual practitioner imposes on herself or himself as a matter of personal professional accountability' (ICN, 1997, cited in Pyne, 1998, p. 252). That, and only that, is what I now regard as self-regulation. For the remainder, I prefer to speak simply of professional regulation, since other stakeholders must be involved in the process if it is to have any credibility either now or in future years.

What hazards must be avoided?

On this matter the ICN text has a succinct answer. It states that 'Regulatory systems should provide and be limited to those controls necessary to achieve their objectives.' In other words, both too little regulation and too much regulation can be harmful to the public interest: the former where it is concerned only with what is required for initial qualification and entry to practice but exerts no influence beyond that point; the latter where it becomes task- or activity-focused and so limits opportunities for innovations in practice, imposes inappropriate limitations on practice and does not take account of the benefits that accrue from overlapping scopes of practice between different health professionals.

Just as a system founded on either too little or too much regulation is a hazard to be avoided, so also is one that does not achieve coordination between the parts. Whether the various component parts of regulation are the responsibility of one organization or several, if they are not properly coordinated, efficient and generally 'fit for purpose', they will fail to deliver.

By the same token, it is important to construct a system that not only addresses local needs, but also fosters professional identity and mobility, providing the opportunity for registered practitioners to practise not only with different employers, but also in different countries. It is for this reason that any form of institutional licensure that is, a system of preparation and licensure that is acceptable to one employer only, is to be avoided.

How to ensure fairness, justice and opportunities for the regulated

In terms of opportunities, a system that pays attention to detail needs to be established and constructed so as to equip the individual to achieve eligibility to practise in organizations or jurisdictions other than their own. As for fairness and justice, while never forgetting the prime purpose for which any profession is regulated – the public interest – and ensuring that this is not jeopardized, the regulatory system should incorporate features that serve to make practitioners confident. They will not feel that confidence or have the feeling that the processes of their regulatory body are fair and just if they are exposed to the risk of being made the scapegoat for the failures of the institution in which they work. They will feel confident if they are satisfied that, when honouring their obligations under their profession's codes of conduct and/or ethics, and exposing actions or omissions that are against the public interest, whether on the part of an individual or an institution, they can act without fear of recrimination.

Conclusion

I have long been, and remain, a passionate believer in professional regulation. I am convinced that it is important that any occupational group of people who treat and care for individuals who are vulnerable, or at times anxious or dependent, be subjected to an effective form of regulation. But to be effective that regulation must be, and must be seen to be, appropriate in all respects.

It must be based on a sound set of principles. It must be constructed so as to be appropriate for the particular country and its population. It must encompass preparation for practice, the requirements for continuation in practice, a means by which to monitor the continuing 'fitness for purpose' of individuals in changing circumstances, and a fair and just system through which, in the public interest, the right to practise can be removed or suspended.

It must have at its heart an organization both empowered and willing to use its accumulated evidence to engage in policy debate and development, the purpose of which is to ensure that good practitioners are supported in practice by effective systems.

The journey I have travelled has seen me move away from a position where I argued that this could only be achieved by a regulatory body with a membership drawn predominantly from within the profession to one that accepts that the reverse can prove more effective and result in greater public confidence. In either set of circumstances, it must be right for those who do serve society as members of professional regulatory bodies to recognize that they are not unique fountains of knowledge and wisdom, and that if they are sensible they draw a wide range of 'others' into their deliberations and decision-making.

Professional regulation matters. It matters to members of the profession, to governments and to employers. But most of all it matters to those who depend on professional practitioners and expect them to be truly accountable. Therefore, whatever system is in place or is proposed for the future, if it fails to ensure that the profession's corporate accountability to that group is fully honoured, it is missing the point. Ask yourself, 'Does the regulatory system where I practise nursing satisfy that criterion?' And if the answer is anything less than a very positive and enthusiastic 'Yes', then ask yourself what *you* intend doing to bring about change.

References

International Council of Nurses (ICN) (1997) *International Council of Nurses on Regulation: Towards 21st Century Models*, Geneva: ICN.

National Consumer Council (1999) *Self-Regulation of Professionals in Health Care*, London: NCC.

Pyne, R.H. (1998) *Professional discipline in nursing, midwifery and health visiting*, 3rd edn, Oxford: Blackwell Science.

Pyne, R.H. (2000) 'Professional regulation: shaken but not stirred', *Consumer Policy Review*, **10** (5), September/October, London: Consumers' Association.

World Health Organization (1995) *Renewing the Health-for-All Strategy. Elaboration of a Policy for Equity, Solidarity and Health*, Consultation Document, Geneva: WHO.

Index